Nuclear Cardiology Study Guide

Andrzej Moniuszko • B. Adrian Kesala

Nuclear Cardiology Study Guide

A Technologist's Review for Passing
Specialty Certification Exams

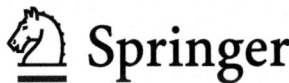 Springer

Andrzej Moniuszko, MD
Department of Radiology
Presence Resurrection Medical Center
Chicago, IL, USA

B. Adrian Kesala, MD
Department of Radiology
Staff Radiologist Presence Resurrection
Medical Center
Chicago, IL, USA

ISBN 978-1-4614-8644-2   ISBN 978-1-4614-8645-9 (eBook)
DOI 10.1007/978-1-4614-8645-9
Springer New York Heidelberg Dordrecht London

Library of Congress Control Number: 2013947921

Printed on acid-free paper

Springer is part of Springer Science+Business Media (www.springer.com)

*I would like to dedicate this work to
my current and past coworkers from the
Nuclear Medicine Department at Presence
Health in Chicago—Sandra Jennings,
Kathleen Tiffin, Anjum Ahmed†,
Marilyn Biel, Michele Strom,
Nisha Varghese, Komal Desai,
Sharon Nyczak, and Brett Nemer
for the willingness to share knowledge
and experience.*

Andrzej Moniuszko, CNMT, ARRT (N),
NCT, PET

This work is dedicated to my wife Larissa

B. Adrian Kesala, MD

Preface

Nuclear Cardiology Study Guide is the third publication in the series of nuclear medicine guides written in question and answer format. All three books—*Nuclear Medicine Technology, PET and PET/CT,* and *Nuclear Cardiology*—collectively provide comprehensive knowledge and cover a broad spectrum of problems involving the application of radioactive substances in the diagnosis and treatment of disease.

This book is designed for technologists, practitioners, students, and trainees in medical imaging to serve as a practical tool to study multiple aspects of nuclear cardiology. It was written and reviewed by individuals who have a wide range of nuclear medicine expertise: a practicing nuclear medicine physician, a nuclear medicine college teacher, and an experienced nuclear medicine technologist. A broad assembly of authors and contributors, with different nuclear medicine experiences, provides an array of problems that technologists and practitioners can, and will, encounter in everyday practice. Some of the questions are easy, and some of them are not. In either case, the book is not designed to test the reader's knowledge. Rather, it should be viewed as tool to learn and deepen knowledge of nuclear cardiology. It is said that a picture is worth a 1,000 words. Our book includes a variety of images, graphics, and diagrams. It is our hope that these illustrations will help the reader to get to the bottom of the problem and come up with the right solution quickly.

The book is divided into four chapters and three appendices. We kick off the book with a chapter on test-taking strategies, which is designed to equip readers with practical tools and methods to successfully navigate through the multiple-choice exam. It was written by a recent Master of Business Administration graduate, a GED Chief Examiner, and an instructor with a Master of Arts in philosophy; their knowledge and hands-on experience provide readers with valuable insider tips.

Chapters 2, 3, and 4 contain the test problems. Each test includes multiple-choice questions, with a total of more than 600 problems. The chapters are organized in three levels of complexity, from the easiest to the most difficult. Generally, tagging questions as easy or difficult is a tricky matter and highly subjective. Nevertheless, for learning purposes, the proposed classification is beneficial for readers. Each chapter is a separate entity with answers and short explanations included. This approach works like building blocks, in which the completion of the first test will prepare the reader to progress to the second test, and so on.

Appendices A and B offer a list of commonly used abbreviations and a glossary of terms which are encountered in everyday nuclear medicine practice and beyond. The abbreviations and the glossary can appear as either too short or simply too long. Some readers will find the included terms as "unnecessary"; some readers will not find the abbreviation for which they are looking. One size never fits all, and thus the subjective choices, as is our selection, are not perfect. Use it to your advantage. There is enough space between the lines, and in the margins, to add or modify as to your own preferences. Understanding the acronyms will pay off in the long run; simply being able to decode it will be short lived. Therefore, a thorough review of the abbreviations and glossary before the examinations can be very helpful and highly suggested. Appendix C offers a list of updated, useful Web sites to refresh knowledge or to learn new skills.

The collection of problems in this book mirrors the exam content as provided by National Medicine Technology Certification Board (NMTCB). The questions cover topics in radiation safety, radionuclides, and instrumentation, to name a few. The reader should never be discouraged when the type of "never heard of" or "it is over my head" problem is encountered. We advise readers to go through these questions carefully and answer diligently—you will be surprised how much you already know and how much you still can learn. Both factors serve as great motivators. Learning should be fun, entertaining, and contagious. Nuclear medicine is a challenging and rapidly evolving field of medicine, and the only way to keep pace with its development is through continuous learning. Nuclear cardiology procedures that were popular in the 1970s are no longer performed, and many new radiotracers and procedures have since been successfully introduced. The integration of molecular imaging not only demonstrates a significant paradigm shift for the specialty but guarantees that nuclear medicine will be a major part of medical practice for the conceivable future.

Be a part of this exciting journey. Make learning fun, and make it a habit—this is the kind of addiction you can afford. The benefits are overwhelming. You can receive the 24 continuing education credit hours, keep your professional license, and, some would say—most importantly—meet your superiors' expectations. You can read, you can study, you can investigate, and you can challenge yourself and others. Best of all you can exceed…your own expectations. The choice is yours.

Again, it is beyond the scope of words to express my appreciation to Prof. Joanne Metler, Coordinator of Nuclear Medicine Technology Program, College of DuPage, IL, for her patience in reviewing the manuscript. Her insight, helpful criticism, suggestions, and insistence on clarity, accuracy, and consistency deserve nothing but my sincere gratitude. I was fortunate enough to be her student, and

I will always appreciate both her deep knowledge of nuclear medicine and her wonderful generosity of spirit. Hope your retirement is everything you expect it to be and much more.

We would also like to thank George Chang, PACS Coordinator, Presence Health, and Todd Monis, Director of Cardiac and Interventional Services, Presence Health, for their instrumental help in preparing clinical images used in this book.

Chicago, IL, USA   Andrzej Moniuszko, CNMT, ARRT (N), NCT, PET
                                                     B. Adrian Kesala, MD

About the Authors

Andrzej Moniuszko, Nuclear Medicine Technologist
Andrzej Moniuszko received an MD degree in 1977 from Medical University in Bialystok, Poland. In 1995 he moved to the USA and two years later passed all exams required by the United States Medical Licensing Examination (USMLE). Given that he was not accepted to the Residency program of his choice and with the goal of furthering his medical career, he completed a Nuclear Medicine Technology Program in College of DuPage, Glen Ellyn, IL. He works as a Nuclear Medicine Technologist in Presence Resurrection Medical Center, Chicago, IL, and holds CNMT, ARRT (N), PET, and NCT certification.

B. Adrian Kesala, MD
Medical Degree: University of Navarra in Spain; Residencies in Diagnostic Radiology, and Nuclear Medicine at Northwestern University, Chicago.
Board certification: American Board of Radiology, American Board of Nuclear Medicine, and Certification of Special Competence in Nuclear Radiology. Former Assistant Professor of Radiology Northwestern University; Senior Attending in Radiology and Director of Nuclear Medicine at Presence Resurrection Medical Center, Chicago.

Contents

Contributors

Beata M. Boies, MA DeKalb Community Unit School District, DeKalb, IL, USA

Josh J. Boies, BS GED Chief Examiner, Geneva, IL, USA

Daryll M. Dickson, RT Cath Lab, Presence Resurrection Medical Center, Chicago, IL, USA

B. Adrian Kesala, MD Department of Radiology, Presence Resurrection Medical Center, Chicago, IL, USA

Natalia Massingill Cardiology, Presence Resurrection Medical Center, Chicago, IL, USA

Andrzej Moniuszko, CNMT, ARRT (N), PET, NCT Department of Radiology, Presence Resurrection Medical Center, Chicago, IL, USA

Marta L. Moniuszko, MBA Aon Hewitt, Lincolnshire, IL, USA

Sabina J. Moniuszko, PTA Department of Physical Therapy, Claremont Hanover Park, Hanover Park, IL, USA

Purvish Patel, RT Department of Radiology, Presence Resurrection Medical Center, Chicago, IL, USA

Chapter 1
Tackling the Multiple-Choice Test

Andrzej Moniuszko, Josh J. Boies, and Beata M. Boies

First of all, congratulations! You are almost ready to take one of the most rewarding and challenging multiple-choice tests. The Nuclear Cardiology specialty exam for a technologist is administered by the Nuclear Medicine Technology Certification Board (NMTCB). First of all, you should visit the Web site: http://www.nmtcb.org/specialty/cardiology.php and familiarize yourself with the test information provided; you will find the information on this site very useful. The NCT exam is now available "on demand." When you are approved, you can choose the date and location for your test..

Multiple choice is the most common test format for standardized tests and is efficient and effective way to measure a wide range of knowledge, skills, attitudes, and abilities. These questions are easier on your recall because they only require you to recognize the correct answer. However, well-designed multiple-choice questions can be difficult; dealing with shades of meaning, conflicting information, appropriate conclusions can make these questions very challenging. Remember that multiple-choice questions require you to choose the best answer, not the correct one.

A. Moniuszko, ARRT (N), PET, NCT. (✉)
Department of Radiology, Staff Radiologist, Presence Resurrection Medical Center, 7435 West Talcott Avenue, Chicago, Cook County, IL 60631, USA
e-mail: mdandy52@yahoo.com

J.J. Boies, BS
GED Chef Examiner, Regional Office of Education, 210 South 6th Street, Geneva, Kane County, IL 60139, USA

B.M. Boies, MA
DeKalb Community Unit School District, 901 South 4th Street, DeKalb, IL 60115, USA

A. Moniuszko and B.A. Kesala, *Nuclear Cardiology Study Guide: A Technologist's Review for Passing Specialty Certification Exams*, DOI 10.1007/978-1-4614-8645-9_1, © Springer Science+Business Media New York 2014

1

A multiple-choice test is composed of three elements: stem, options, and distractors. The stem is the basic problem. The stem may be either a question or an incomplete statement. Options are the list of responses available. The list contains one correct answer. The remaining responses act as the distractors. The distractors are designed to appear as plausible answers.

You need to know and read all the directions carefully, know if each question has one or more correct options, know if you are going to be penalized for guessing, and know how much time is being allowed to complete the test.

Let's lay down the different methods and strategies for taking the multiple-choice test.

First, try covering the list of responses with your hand, read the stem carefully, and answer the question before looking at the possible choices. By doing so, you will not be negatively influenced or confused by the available choices. Pick the response which best matches your initial answer. Second, read the stem thoroughly (you can write down the important words), determine what is being asked, and then read all the answers carefully. Compare each choice to what you think is the correct answer, eliminate the obviously incorrect answers, and choose your answer from the remaining options. Another useful approach is to read the stem together with each of the options, one by one. Treat each combination as if it was a True/False question. If the combined statement is false, you can eliminate that option; if it appears to be correct mark it as a possible answer. Repeat this for all alternatives.

For questions that are more complicated, try to simplify the stem and rephrase the answers. Using this strategy both the stem and the options will be clearer, and they will make more sense to you. This makes the question more manageable. When you answer difficult questions eliminate options you know are incorrect; have reservations about answers that are totally unfamiliar to you. If you know that multiple options are correct, the statement, "All of the above," is the strongest possibility. If none of the choices available to you match your predetermined answer, you can use one of the following techniques to narrow down to the probable answer: Responses containing phrases such as "All of the above" or "None of the above" are also more likely to be true. However, you must be careful. Read all of the preceding responses and ensure all or none of them apply. Be cautious of trap words such as "never," "every," "always," "only," and "completely." Read the alternatives containing these words very thoroughly. Keep in mind that options with absolute phrases suggest that the statement is always true, which is rarely correct. On the other hand, words such as "might," "generally," "some," "usually," and "often" are clues that the answer might be correct.

It is a good and advised practice to answer the easy questions first. If you don't know the solution use your knowledge to narrow down the possibilities, tag each item appropriately, and then go back later and reattempt to find the answers. Remember, the entire test is full of hints, and information contained in one part may help you in another. Keep in mind, usually your first choice is the correct one. Unless you determine based on information further along in the test or you are certain you misread the stem or the alternatives, you should not change your answer.

If all of the above fails, guess, but do not guesstimate until you have eliminated all of the definitely incorrect options. When you are forced to guess, always make a knowledge-based guess—use hints from questions you know to answer questions you do not; if you have used all you know to narrow down the possibilities, and you still cannot decide between two or more choices, you should use your knowledge of probability.

And yes, change your first answers when you are sure of the correction, or if other clues in the test cue you to change. You are allowed to review your choices and change any answer before submitting the test.

Each test administrator offers a brief test tutorial before the examination with sample questions. These are designed to help you familiarize yourself with the test process and the format of the questions. What if the test administrator is unprofessional and your test anxiety begins to grow? Do not worry. Most of these people are here to help you. Yes, you may be treated poorly during the check-in process. You may be told to empty your pockets, leave your phone and wallet, roll up your sleeves, etc. Do not let this bother you; these are precautions to prevent test-takers from cheating. Remember, you are well prepared to pass the multiple-choice test. In the next chapter, we will be learning more about how to deal with test anxiety. The nervousness you feel is likely to increase as you near your test exam date and it will usually peak during the actual examination. Therefore, it is important we look into the arsenal of anxiety-fighting tools.

Dealing with the Test Anxiety

Preparation, both mental and physical, is said to be the number one remedy for text anxiety. There is a myriad of literature on the subject of studying methods. Having gone as far as you have in your life, we trust you must have developed a good study technique that has carried you this far. Let's review study preparations that will help you to deal with test anxiety.

Build a study plan. You know what works for you, build the strategy accordingly. Be realistic and remember, as Dwight D. Eisenhower once said about preparing for battle, "Plans are worthless, but planning is indispensable." Also know that your plans can change and be prepared to handle changes. Never procrastinate and always manage your study time wisely. The study guide you hold in your hand is designed to help you navigate through the preparation.

Here are a few study tips:

Have a positive attitude and at the same time, eliminate any negative thoughts.

Arrange your schedule to minimize any outside distractions. You should have a designated study area, preferably in a secluded, quiet, and well-lit place.

Determine the part of the material you are going to study and for how long. Have everything ready and within reach. Remove everything that is not related to that particular section.

If you catch yourself day dreaming or losing concentration, switch to a different
   study area or subject.

Take breaks. You can stretch, take a brisk walk or eat a snack.

Stop studying when you are feeling tired or you are simply no longer productive.

Exercise in the days leading to the exam. It will significantly reduce your stress level.

Approach the exam with confidence.

Get a good night of sleep the night before exam.

Allow yourself plenty of time to arrive at the test center and be sure to get there early.

Relax just before the exam. Don't try to do any last minute review.

Do not go to the exam with an empty stomach.

During the test stay relaxed and confident.

Be comfortable but alert.

Preview the test and answer the questions in a strategic order.

Get right to the point.

Reserve 10 % of your test time for review.

Do not panic when other test-takers finish before you. It is not a race.

Dress comfortably, preferably in layers so you are able to adjust your attire to the
   temperature inside the testing center.

Being mentally and physically prepared is bound to eliminate the majority of the
test-related anxiety. However, there is always a small percentage of anxiety that will
be present in a high stakes environment. Accept it, and it will actually help you stay
alert and sharpen your mental reflexes. On the day of the examination remain
relaxed. Take a moment for yourself to perform a couple of slow-breathing exer-
cises. Simultaneously, visualize yourself at a peaceful place. During the test, con-
centrate only on questions. Your goal is to answer them correctly. That is all that
matters. The best tennis players win because they never let the ball out of their eye
sight. Follow their winning practices. After the examination is completed, reward
yourself for your hard work.

Thomas A. Edison once said: "Many of life's failures are people who did not
realize how close they were to success when they gave up." Stay focused and never
give up. Good luck!

References

Blackey R. So many choices, so little time: strategies for understanding and taking multiple-choice
   exams in history. Hist Teach. 2009;43(1):53–66.

Gloe D. Study habits and test-taking tips. Dermatol Nurs. 1999;11:493–9.

Kubistant T. Test performance: the neglected skill. Education. 2001;102(1):53–5.

NMTCB. Cardiology exam information. Test taking power strategies. New York, NY: Learning
   Express; 2007. http://www.nmtcb.org/specialty/cardiology.php

Study guides and strategies. Overcoming test anxiety. http://www.studygs.net/tstprp8.htm.
   Accessed 12 Sep 2010.

Taking multiple choice exams. http://www.uwec.edu/geography/Ivogeler/multiple.htm. Accessed
   20 Sep 2010.

Chapter 2
Practice Test #1: Difficulty Level—Easy

Andrzej Moniuszko and B. Adrian Kesala

Questions

1. The first-pass myocardial extraction fraction of Tl-201 is in the range of:
   A. 95 %
   B. 85 %
   C. 75 %
   D. 65 %

2. Tl-201 myocardial imaging, when compared with Tc-99 m-based tracers:
   A. Creates less soft tissue attenuation
   B. Produces improved image quality
   C. Produces improved image contrast
   D. Creates less liver and gut activity

3. On the SPECT 17-segment model, myocardial perfusion is graded within each segment on a scale of:
   A. 0–4
   B. 0–8
   C. 1–4
   D. 1–8

Answers to Test #1 begin on page 44

A. Moniuszko, ARRT (N), PET, NCT. (✉) • B.A. Kesala, M.D.
Department of Radiology, Staff Radiologist, Presence Resurrection Medical Center,
7435 West Talcott Avenue, Chicago, Cook County, IL 60631, USA
e-mail: mdandy52@yahoo.com

A. Moniuszko and B.A. Kesala, *Nuclear Cardiology Study Guide: A Technologist's Review for Passing Specialty Certification Exams*, DOI 10.1007/978-1-4614-8645-9_2, © Springer Science+Business Media New York 2014

4. The physical half-life of O-15 is:
   A. 63 s
   B. 124 s
   C. 248 s
   D. 496 s

5. An immune inflammatory process, which over decades, results in the heart's arterial narrowing, is called:
   A. Arrhythmia
   B. Coronary artery disease
   C. Myocardial infarction
   D. Unstable angina

6. Substantial tracer uptake observed throughout the lung fields after stress, that is not present at rest, indicates a diagnosis of:
   A. Bronchial asthma
   B. Cardiac arrhythmia
   C. Lung carcinoma
   D. Severe ischemia

7. An indirect coronary vasodilator that works by increasing intravascular adenosine levels is called:
   A. Adenosine
   B. Dipyridamole
   C. Dobutamine
   D. Regadenoson

8. A photoelectric method allowing the monitoring of the degree of oxygen saturation of the blood hemoglobin is called:
   A. Absorptiometry
   B. Oximetry
   C. Spectrophotometry
   D. Sphygmomanometry

9. Which of the following tracers has ~ 50 % myocardial clearance at 6 h?
   A. Tc-99m sestamibi
   B. Tc-99m teboroxime
   C. Tc-99m tetrofosmin
   D. Thallium-201

10. The maximum heart rate (HR) can be estimated utilizing the following formula:
    A. HR = 220 + age (in years)
    B. HR = 220 − age (in years)
    C. HR = (220 + age in years) × 0.85
    D. HR = (220 − age in years) × 0.85

11. The sum of segmental scores from the rest images (the summed rest score, SRS) represents the extent of:
    A. Hibernation
    B. Ischemia
    C. Infarction
    D. Viability

12. The nuclear cardiology procedure during which a dynamic bolus of radioactivity is imaged as it quickly transits through different chambers of the heart and lungs is called:
    A. Equilibrium gated radionuclide angiography
    B. First-pass radionuclide angiography
    C. Gated single photon emission computed tomography
    D. Infarct avid imaging study

13. Which of the following approaches has NOT been effective in reducing the impact of breast tissue attenuation on the specificity of myocardial perfusion?
    A. Reviewing of the cine display
    B. Performing delay imaging
    C. The use of Tc-99 m-based agents with SPECT imaging
    D. The use of electrocardiography (ECG) gating

14. During PET acquisition the emitted positron travels in the tissues until it collides with a/an:
    A. Electron
    B. Neutron
    C. Positron
    D. Proton

15. The Coronary flow reserve (CFR) is defined as the ratio of:
    A. Stress-to-rest perfusion
    B. Rest-to-delay rest perfusion
    C. Stress-to-delay stress perfusion
    D. Rest-to-stress perfusion

16. In healthy patients, the following hemodynamic changes are observed during exercise EXCEPT:
    A. Total calculated peripheral resistance decreases
    B. Oxygen extraction increases
    C. Diastolic blood pressure decreases
    D. Skeletal muscle blood flow is increased

17. Which of the following SPECT filters has NO selectable parameters?
    A. The Butterworth filter
    B. The ramp filter
    C. The Parzen filter
    D. The Hanning filter

18. The ECG silver chloride electrodes are covered with a fluid column in order to:
    A. Avoid direct metal to skin contact
    B. Prevent skin infection
    C. Reduce skin resistance
    D. Remove skin oil

19. The MPI artifacts described as falsely "hotter" or falsely "cold" cardiac regions are caused by:
    A. Patient motion
    B. Gating error
    C. Extracardiac activity
    D. Breast attenuation

20. The metabolic equivalent task (MET)—a unit of oxygen uptake in a sitting, resting person is corresponding to:
    A. 3.5 ml O2/kg/h of body weight
    B. 3.5 ml O2/kg/min of body weight
    C. 7.0 ml O2/kg/h of body weight
    D. 7.0 ml O2/kg/min of body weight

21. Thallium clearance from normal myocardium with high thallium activity, when compared with clearance from ischemic myocardium, is:
    A. Dose dependent
    B. Faster
    C. Slower
    D. The same

22. In patients undergoing pharmacologic stress test with adenosine, adjunctive low-level exercise is effective in:
    A. Lowering patient radiation exposure
    B. Improving imaging characteristics
    C. Reducing personnel radiation exposure
    D. Lessening motion artifacts

23. The extent and severity of stress-induced ischemia is represented by:
   A. The summed rest score (SRS)
   B. The summed stress score (SSS)
   C. The summed difference score (SDS)
   D. All of the above

24. Which of the following PET techniques are employed to assess myocardial viability?
   A. N-13 ammonia as a metabolic marker of glucose use and FDG as a perfusion tracer
   B. N-13 ammonia and FDG as perfusion tracers
   C. N-13 ammonia and FDG as metabolic marker of glucose use
   D. N-13 ammonia as a perfusion tracer and FDG as a metabolic marker of glucose use

25. The substance deposited in the walls of the coronary arteries that is made up of a complex mixture of fats, including cholesterol and cell debris is called:
   A. Atheroma
   B. Calcium
   C. Cholesterol
   D. Lipoma

26. In a typical gated SPECT acquisition, the frame in the middle of the cardiac cycle represents the event called:
   A. End-diastolic
   B. End-systolic
   C. Mid-diastolic
   D. Mid-systolic

27. A 58-year-old woman presents to her primary care physician with complaints of atypical chest pain over last few days. She currently is asymptomatic and has no significant past medical, family, or social history. The electrocardiogram (Fig. 2.1) shows:
   A. Atrial fibrillation
   B. Electronic ventricular pacemaker
   C. Normal sinus rhythm
   D. Ventricular bigeminy

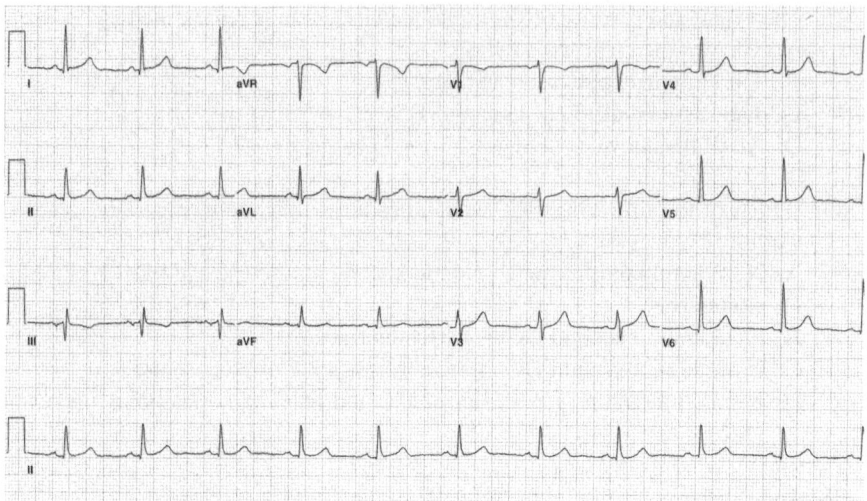

Fig. 2.1 Electrocardiogram

28. Optimizing selection of patients with heart failure whose symptoms and natural history may improve after revascularization is the goal of performing:
    A. Coronary angiography
    B. Stress echocardiography
    C. Stress MPI study
    D. Viability study

29. All of the following statements correctly describe findings from a direct comparison of SPECT MPI with PET MPI EXCEPT:
    A. PET has shown significantly improved normalcy rate
    B. PET has shown significantly improved sensitivity
    C. SPECT has shown a superior diagnostic performance when subanalyzed for gender
    D. SPECT ability to identify multivessel ischemia was significantly lower

30. The exercise stress test should be stopped if:
    A. There are technical difficulties in monitoring systolic blood pressure
    B. 1 mm of ST depression is present
    C. Arterial blood pressure is 200/110
    D. Systolic blood pressure drops by 15 mmHg

31. The counts distribution of all short-axis slices displayed in concentric rings is called:
    A. A bull's eye
    B. A counts profile
    C. A planogram
    D. A sinogram

32. During equilibrium gated radionuclide angiography (ERNA), images are acquired after the administered radioactivity has equilibrated in the:
    A. Endocardium
    B. Lymphatic space
    C. Myocardium
    D. Vascular space

33. The term incremental value of SPECT MPI implies that perfusion imaging data provide information on the natural history, risk, and outcomes that are:
    A. Additive to information from more available or less expensive tests
    B. More valuable than information from more available or less expensive tests
    C. Contradictive to information from more available or less expensive tests
    D. Less valuable than information from more available or less expensive tests

34. A strontium Sr-82 generator can be used for up to:
    A. 1 week
    B. 1 month
    C. 6 months
    D. 1 year

35. Peak exercise in normal individuals produces an increase in myocardial oxygen demand and .... increase in myocardial blood flow:
    A. A twofold
    B. A twofold to threefold
    C. A threefold to fourfold
    D. A fourfold to fivefold

36. Which of the following exercise protocols is most frequently used to assess cardiovascular reserve?
    A. Dynamic exercise
    B. Isometric exercise
    C. Resistive exercise
    D. Static exercise

37. Patients scheduled for a pharmacological stress test with Lexiscan should be instructed to avoid consumption of any products containing methylxanthines for at least:
    A. 3 h
    B. 6 h
    C. 12 h
    D. 24 h

38. The proportion of tracer removed from the blood as it passes through the myocardium is called:
    A. First-pass extraction fraction
    B. Ejection fraction
    C. Coronary flow reserve
    D. Myocardial blood flow

39. Gated single photon emission computed tomography (GSPECT) is not suitable for accurate right ventricular function measurement because the RV:
    A. Is not visualized
    B. Is not adequately visualized
    C. Is attenuated by the liver
    D. Is attenuated by the spleen

40. The room temperature of the treadmill stress testing area should be between:
    A. 55° and 63° F
    B. 64° and 72° F
    C. 73° and 80° F
    D. 80° and 85° F

41. Thallium washes out of the myocardium at a rate dependent on:
    A. Injected dose
    B. Local myocardial perfusion
    C. Local ejection fraction
    D. Blood pressure

42. During a typical stress Tc-99m tetrofosmin study, imaging begins:
    A. 5 min after the exercise stress injection and 10–15 min after the pharmacological stress injection
    B. 5 min after the exercise stress injection and 20–30 min after the pharmacological stress injection
    C. 10 min after the exercise stress injection and 20–30 min after the pharmacological stress injection
    D. 10 min after the exercise stress injection and 30–45 min after the pharmacological stress injection

43. All of the following approaches have been used in high-speed SPECT technology EXCEPT:
    A. Novel image reconstruction algorithm
    B. Slip ring technology
    C. Solid-state detector columns with cadmium zinc telluride
    D. Wide-angle tungsten collimators

44. Which of the following protocols stimulating maximal F-18 FDG uptake is based on the simultaneous infusion of insulin and glucose?
    A. Euglycemic hypoinsulinemic clamp protocol
    B. Euglycemic hyperinsulinemic clamp protocol
    C. Hypoglycemic hyperinsulinemic clamp protocol
    D. Hypoglycemic hypoinsulinemic clamp protocol

45. Viable myocardial tissue is NOT present in:
    A. Infarcted myocardium
    B. Ischemic myocardium
    C. Stunned myocardium
    D. Hibernating myocardium

46. Visual comparison of MPI stress and rest displays revealing a perfusion defect that is seen on stress but not on rest images describes:
    A. Normal myocardium
    B. Ischemic myocardium
    C. Scarred myocardium
    D. Stunned myocardium

47. Lexiscan (regadenoson) is contraindicated in patients with:
    A. Asthma
    B. Hypovolemia
    C. Pericarditis
    D. Sinus node dysfunction

48. The areas of ECG electrode application are rubbed with an alcohol-saturated pad to remove from the skin:
    A. Bacteria
    B. Hair
    C. Oil
    D. Sweat

49. Tl-201 emits 80 keV of photon energy and has a physical half-life of:
    A. 53 h
    B. 63 h
    C. 73 h
    D. 83 h

50. The Bruce protocol begins with:
    A. A treadmill speed of 1.7 mph and a grade of 0°
    B. A treadmill speed of 1.7 mph and a grade of 10°
    C. A treadmill speed of 3.4 mph and a grade of 0°
    D. A treadmill speed of 3.4 mph and a grade of 10°

51. Tl-201 compared with the 99mTc-based agents:
    A. Offers improved performance in patients with large breasts
    B. Offers improved performance in obese patients
    C. Delivers a higher radiation dose
    D. Allows the option of higher quality gated images

52. During a GSPECT acquisition, one cardiac cycle is represented by the:
    A. P–Q interval
    B. P–R interval
    C. R–R interval
    D. R–T interval

53. All of the following are examples of MPI automated quantitative analysis systems incorporated into SPECT camera-computer equipment EXCEPT:
    A. Cedars QPS
    B. 4D-MSPECT
    C. McKesson Practice Choice Software
    D. Emory Toolbox

54. Which of the following are the physical characteristics of the positron emitted by Rb-82?
    A. Energy of 511 keV and average range of 2.8 mm
    B. Energy of 3.15 MeV and average range of 2.8 mm
    C. Energy of 3.15 MeV and average range of 0.22 mm
    D. Energy of 511 keV and average range of 0.22 mm

55. The typical ejection fraction (EF) of the left ventricle is approximately:
    A. 100 %
    B. 87 %
    C. 58 %
    D. 29 %

56. During the exercise stress test, the heart rate, blood pressure, and ECG should be recorded (select three):
    A. At the beginning of each stage of exercise
    B. At the onset of an ischemic response
    C. Immediately after stopping exercise
    D. Every minute in the stage 3
    E. In the middle of each stage of exercise
    F. The end of each stage of exercise

57. An adenosine injection is contraindicated in individuals with:
    A. Atrial fibrillation
    B. Bigeminy
    C. Pacemaker
    D. Third-degree AV block

58. All of the following diagnostic procedures are available on PET-CT scanners equipped with multislice CT EXCEPT:
    A. Coronary calcium measurement
    B. Coronary angiography
    C. Doppler echocardiography
    D. PET viability study

59. Gated single photon emission computed tomography (GSPECT) acquisition starts with the R wave on the ECG which corresponds to the:
    A. End-diastole
    B. End-systole
    C. Mid-diastole
    D. Mid-systole

60. The number of correct findings on a MPI test, regardless of whether the patient has CAD, describes the diagnostic test:
    A. Accuracy
    B. Reproducibility
    C. Sensitivity
    D. Specificity

61. Which of the following patients are the best candidates for gated SPECT studies?
    A. Patients with atrial fibrillation
    B. Patients with premature atrial contractions
    C. Patients with premature ventricular contractions
    D. Patients with sinus rhythm

62. Which of the following statements correctly describe properties of Tc-99m versus Tl-201 as radionuclide tracers for myocardial imaging?
    A. Tc-99m has a higher emission energy and a longer half-life than Tl-201
    B. Tc-99m has a higher emission energy and a shorter half-life than Tl-201
    C. Tc-99m has a lower emission energy and a longer half-life than Tl-201
    D. Tc-99m has a lower emission energy and a shorter half-life than Tl-201

63. Which of the following factors/conditions can be a reason of a false positive MPI study?
    A. Balanced ischemia
    B. Suboptimal level of exercise
    C. Left bundle branch block
    D. Patient on nitrates

64. The most frequently used clinical myocardial perfusion PET agent is:
    A. F-18 FDG
    B. Rb-82
    C. Tc 99 m-sestamibi
    D. Tl-201

65. Myocardial oxygen consumption (MVO2) is measured in the units of:
    A. ml O2/min per kg
    B. ml O2/min per 100 g
    C. ml O2/h per 100 g
    D. lO2/min per 100 g

66. Tl-201, when compared with technetium 99 m-based myocardial imaging:
    A. Creates less soft tissue attenuation
    B. Produces improved image quality
    C. Produces improved image contrast
    D. Creates less liver and gut activity

67. The most common adverse reaction associated with adenosine administration is/are:
    A. Arrhythmias
    B. Flushing
    C. Hypotension
    D. Paresthesias

68. Heparin and warfarin are:
    A. Antibiotics
    B. Anticoagulants
    C. Antiemetics
    D. Antipyretics

69. The major vasodilators used for pharmacologic radionuclide myocardial perfusion imaging (rMPI) are (select three):
    A. Adenosine
    B. Aggrenox
    C. Atropine
    D. Dipyridamole
    E. Regadenoson

70. Which of the following is absolute contraindication for exercise stress testing?
    A. Acute pulmonary embolism
    B. Left main coronary artery stenosis
    C. Physical impairment
    D. Significant tachyarrhythmias

71. MPI has the greatest diagnostic value for detection of CAD when it is used in patients with:
    A. A very low pretest likelihood of disease
    B. A low pretest likelihood of disease
    C. A moderate pretest likelihood of disease
    D. A high pretest likelihood of disease

72. Tomographic reconstruction theory can be described as:
    A. A 3-dimensional image volume reconstituted from a series of 2-dimensional images
    B. A 3-dimensional image volume reconstituted from a series of 3-dimensional images
    C. A 2-dimensional image volume reconstituted from a series of 2-dimensional images
    D. A 2-dimensional image volume reconstituted from a series of 3-dimensional images

73. Upward creep of the heart observed during SPECT acquisition could be prevented by:
    A. Acquiring gated images
    B. Adjusting patient stress dose
    C. Allowing bed rest before SPECT
    D. Adjusting patient rest dose

74. Beta (+) decay of a nucleus results in emission of a/an:
    A. Electron
    B. Neutron
    C. Positron
    D. Proton

75. Which of the following belongs to the left cardiovascular system (select three)?
    A. The left side of the heart
    B. The pulmonary arteries
    C. The pulmonary veins
    D. The right side of the heart
    E. The systemic arterial system
    F. The venous system

76. Medications such as calcium channel blocking drugs and beta-blockers administered on the day of exercise stress MPI may alter:
    A. The heart rate
    B. The respiration rate
    C. The body temperature
    D. The basic metabolic rate

77. Tomographic reconstruction of projection images produces transaxial images which are:
    A. Perpendicular to the long axis of the patient
    B. Parallel to the long axis of the patient
    C. Horizontal to the long axis of the left ventricle
    D. Vertical to the long axis of the left ventricle

78. How many separated channels does a Foley catheter have?
    A. One
    B. Two
    C. Three
    D. Four

79. The LV ejection fraction (LVEF) measured from the GSPECT 8-frame acquisition when compared to the 16-frame acquisition is:
    A. 3 units lower
    B. 13 units lower
    C. 3 units higher
    D. 13 units higher

80. The myocardial blood flow (MBF) in coronary beds without significant stenosis increases ~threefold with:
    A. Exercise
    B. Dipyridamole
    C. Dobutamine
    D. Regadenoson

81. A vertical change in position of the heart that is usually noticed between the last frame of detector 2 and the first frame of detector 1 is called:
    A. Horizontal shift
    B. Hurricane sign
    C. Upward creep
    D. Star artifact

82. A 51-year-old man presents to the emergency department with sudden onset of palpitations and mild lightheadedness. He had experienced briefer episodes over the last 2 months, but this episode persisted for 4 min. The ECG (Fig. 2.2) shows:
    A. Atrial fibrillation
    B. Electronic ventricular pacemaker
    C. Normal sinus rhythm
    D. Ventricular bigeminy

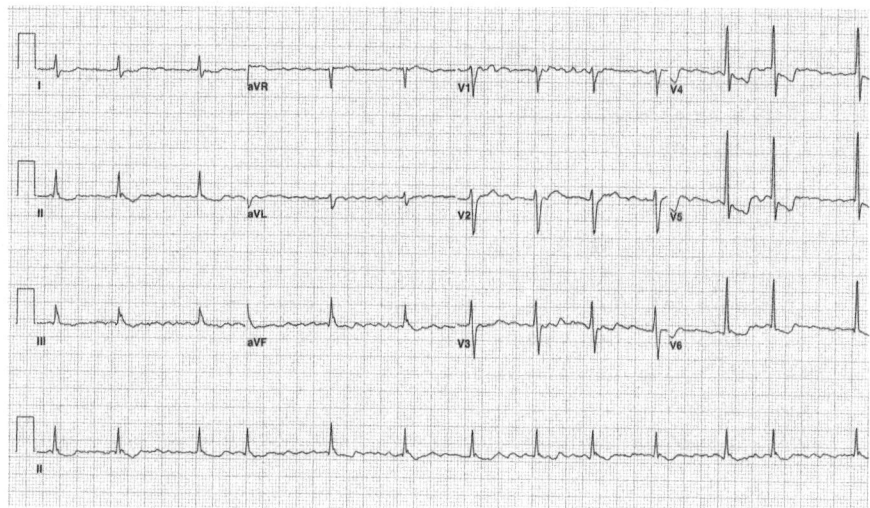

Fig. 2.2 Electrocardiogram

83. Thallium is predominantly cleared by:
    A. The hepatobiliary system
    B. The kidneys
    C. The skin
    D. The respiratory system

84. Glycolysis is the metabolic pathway converting glucose 6-phosphate to:
    A. Acetate
    B. Fructose
    C. Pyruvate
    D. Sucrose

85. The percentage of patients without CAD with a negative test result compared with the total number of patients tested without CAD describes the test:
    A. Specificity
    B. Sensitivity
    C. Accuracy
    D. Reproducibility

86. Activation of adenosine A_2A receptors produces:
    A. Atrioventricular conduction delay
    B. Bronchospasm
    C. Coronary vasodilatation
    D. Tachycardia

87. When performing a pharmacological stress test with Lexiscan, the myocardial perfusion imaging agent should be administered:
    A. 1–5 s before Lexiscan administration
    B. Immediately after Lexiscan injection
    C. Immediately after the saline flush
    D. 10–20 s after the saline flush

88. Which of the following medications are commonly referred to as "blood thinners"?
    A. Antibiotics
    B. Anticoagulants
    C. Antiemetics
    D. Antipyretics

89. The MPI test sensitivity for ischemia is enhanced by getting the patient to perform the exercise portion of the test to a maximal safe level defined as:
    A. The maximal 65 % of age-predicted heart rate is reached
    B. The maximal 75 % of age-predicted heart rate is reached
    C. The maximal 85 % of age-predicted heart rate is reached
    D. The maximal 95 % of age-predicted heart rate is reached

90. According to the ASNC IMAGING GUIDELINES FOR NUCLEAR CARDIOLOGY PROCEDURES, all exercise tests should be limited by:
    A. Patient age
    B. Achieved double product
    C. Achieved 85 % of maximum heart rate
    D. Symptoms

91. In hybrid imaging, an attenuation map represents the degree of photon attenuation and is acquired:
    A. For every patient
    B. Daily
    C. Weekly
    D. For group of patients

92. Chest pain that develops commonly during pharmacologic vasodilator stress testing:
    A. Indicates severe CAD
    B. Indicates poor prognosis
    C. Is a nonspecific finding
    D. Is a marker of vascular reactivity

93. All of the following appropriateness designation for cardiovascular tests are given in the appropriate use criteria (AUC) document EXCEPT:
    A. Appropriate
    B. Uncertain
    C. Expensive
    D. Inappropriate

94. The relative differences in count values between myocardial pixels are displayed in the black and white images as a variation in:
    A. Brightness
    B. Dimension
    C. Shape
    D. Sharpness

95. Uncharacteristic communications between the left and right sides of the heart known as a ventricular septal defect (VSD) initially results in:
    A. Pulmonary hypertension
    B. A R-L shunt
    C. A L-R shunt
    D. A pulmonary embolism

96. Administered dose of which of the following pharmacologic stress agents is NOT weight-adjusted?
    A. Adenosine
    B. Dipyridamole
    C. Dobutamine
    D. Regadenoson

97. Figure 2.3 displays images acquired during routine 32 frames multi-gated acquisition (MUGA) scan. The end diastole image is labeled:
    A. D
    B. C
    C. B
    D. A

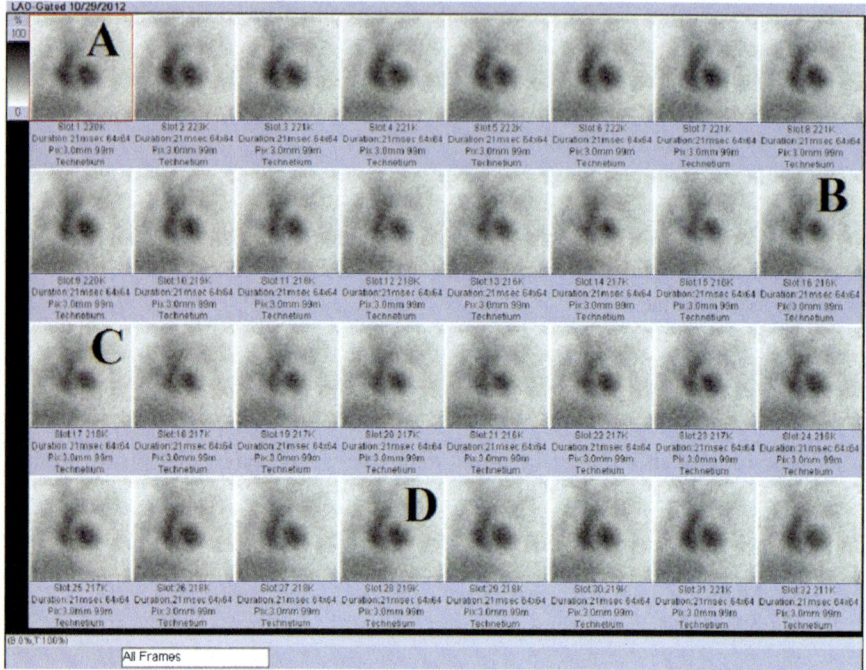

Fig. 2.3 MUGA scan

98. For a trained rescuer performing adult CPR, what do the 2010 American Heart Association (AHA) guidelines for CPR and ECC recommend as the first step in the CPR sequence?
    A. Airway
    B. Breathing
    C. Chest compression
    D. Defibrillation

99. Infusion of intravenous aminophylline antagonizes the effects of:
    A. Atropine
    B. The vasodilator stress agents
    C. The inotropic stress agents
    D. Propranolol

100. With increasing workloads, the normal systolic blood pressure of a healthy person:
    A. Decreases progressively by 20 mmHg/stage
    B. Doesn't change during exercise
    C. Increases progressively to a peak response ranging from 160–200 mmHg
    D. Increases progressively to a peak response ranging from 200–260 mmHg

101. Which of the following MPI protocols provides optimal defect contrast with minimal background activity?
    A. Same day low dose rest, high stress protocol
    B. Same day low dose stress high dose rest protocol
    C. Two-day protocol
    D. Dual-isotope protocol

102. The view comprising oblique tomographic cuts generated by slicing along the short axis perpendicular to the long axis of the left ventricle is called:
    A. Long-axis view
    B. Short-axis view
    C. Vertical long-axis view
    D. Horizontal long-axis view

103. Appropriate use criteria (AUC) assess all of the following aspects of cardio-vascular testing EXCEPT:
    A. When to perform a test
    B. How often to perform a test
    C. How much does a test cost
    D. In whom to perform a test

104. All of the following are cyclotron-produced positron emitters EXCEPT:
    A. F-18
    B. N-13
    C. O-15
    D. Rb-82

105. Conception is unlikely to have happened:
    A. Within the first 10 day of the menstrual cycle
    B. Within 10–15 days of the menstrual cycle
    C. Within 16–20 days of the menstrual cycle
    D. Within 21–25 days of the menstrual cycle

106. Soft tissue attenuation artifacts decrease the diagnostic accuracy of SPECT in myocardial perfusion imaging as a result of increase in:
    A. False positive rate
    B. False negative rate
    C. True positive rate
    D. True negative rate

107. The recommended intravenous dose of Adenoscan for adults is:
    A. 100 mcg/kg/min infused for 6 min
    B. 140 mcg/kg/min infused for 6 min
    C. 100 mcg/kg/min infused for 3 min
    D. 140 mcg/kg/min infused for 3 min

108. The insertion of an intravenous line is suggested for the radiopharmaceutical injection of rest and stress parts of MPI in order to:
    A. Reduce the possibility of an infiltrated dose
    B. Reduce the possibility of motion artifacts
    C. Increase patient comfort
    D. Improve signal-to-noise ratio

109. All of the following parameters can be assessed by performing an exercise stress in conjunction with MPI EXCEPT the patient's:
    A. Functional capacity
    B. Stress-induced electrocardiographic changes
    C. Heart rate recovery
    D. Stress-induced echocardiographic changes

110. A modified Bruce protocol is used for exercise testing in those patients who are:
    A. Assertive
    B. Athletic
    C. Old and frail
    D. Young and strong

111. Which of the following statements describing properties of technetium-based MPI tracers or thallium is CORRECT?
    A. Technetium first-pass myocardial extraction is 85 %, its energy is lower than optimum for current gamma cameras
    B. Thallium first-pass myocardial extraction is 60 %, its energy is lower than optimum for current gamma cameras
    C. Thallium first-pass myocardial extraction is 85 %, its energy results in less scatter and soft tissue attenuation
    D. Technetium first-pass myocardial extraction is 60 %, its energy results in less scatter and soft tissue attenuation

112. The heart responds to dobutamine infusion similarly to the way it responds to:
    A. Adenosine
    B. Dipyridamole
    C. Exercise
    D. Regadenoson

113. An acceptance window of 20 % allows acquiring data from cardiac cycles having a duration within:
    A. ± 20 % of the mean R–R interval
    B. ± 10 % of the mean R–R interval
    C. ± 5 % of the mean R–R interval
    D. ± 2 % of the mean R–R interval

114. Which of the following PET agents is classified as the freely diffusible tracer?
   A. F-18 fluorodeoxyglucose
   B. N-13 ammonia
   C. O-15 water
   D. Rb-82

115. Present guidelines for the treatment of patients with acute myocardial infarction include all of the following options EXCEPT:
   A. Coronary revascularization
   B. Medical therapy
   C. Radiation therapy
   D. Thrombolytic agents

116. Which of the following statements, describing extracardiac incidental findings (ECFs) on nuclear SPECT MPI, is FALSE?
   A. ECFs on nuclear SPECT MPI are common and can be easily identified
   B. ECFs can be small or large and they can be single or multiple
   C. Patients with ECFs may have symptoms that can often mimic cardiac symptoms
   D. There is a significant variability in the incidence of reported ECFs, depending on the reader's skill

117. What is the correct order of injections when a pharmacological stress test with Lexiscan is performed?
   A. Saline flash, Lexiscan, radiotracer, saline flash
   B. Lexiscan, saline flash, radiotracer, saline flash
   C. Radiotracer, saline flash, Lexiscan, saline flash
   D. Radiotracer, saline flash, Lexiscan, saline flash

118. The perfusion–metabolism mismatch pattern—reduced perfusion and preserved metabolism—has been considered the hallmark of:
   A. Hibernating myocardium
   B. Normal myocardium
   C. Scarred myocardium
   D. Stunned myocardium

119. The distribution information obtained by the gated SPECT with Tc-99m-based tracers reflects the perfusion at the time of:
   A. Acquisition
   B. Initial evaluation
   C. Injection
   D. Test termination

120. A measure of the work load of the heart, equal to systolic blood pressure mul-
tiplied by heart rate, is called:
A. The double product
B. The heart rate recovery
C. The metabolic equivalent
D. The predicted heart rate

121. LVEF is derived from the end-diastolic volume (EDV) and the end-systolic
volume (ESV) using the formula:
A. (EDV−ESV)/EDV×100
B. (EDV+ESV)/EDV×100
C. (EDV−ESV)/ESV×100
D. (EDV+ESV)/ESV×100

122. Imaging after Tc-99m sestamibi administration is best done after a brief wait-
ing period to allow for some liver and biliary clearance, but before significant
accumulation of the radiotracer in the:
A. Bladder
B. Stomach
C. Spleen
D. Transverse colon

123. Sestamibi and tetrofosmin are lipid-soluble cationic compounds with first-
pass extraction fractions in the range of:
A. 50 %
B. 60 %
C. 70 %
D. 80 %

124. F-18fluorodeoxyglucose is trapped in the myocyte as:
A. F-18 FDG-6-phosphate
B. F-18 FDG-4-phosphate
C. F-18 FDG-2-phosphate
D. F-18 FDG-1-phosphate

125. The typical stroke volume (SV) of the left ventricle is approximately:
A. 35 ml
B. 70 ml
C. 140 ml
D. 280 ml

126. Which of the following will increase the sensitivity of Tl-201 for detection of viable myocardium?
   A. Applying attenuation correction
   B. Increasing the tracer dose
   C. Obtaining gated images
   D. Reinjecting the tracer

127. What is the recommended intravenous dose of Lexiscan?
   A. 4 ml (0.5 mg regadenoson)
   B. 5 ml (0.2 mg regadenoson)
   C. 5 ml (0.4 mg regadenoson)
   D. 4 ml (0.4 mg regadenoson)

128. After oral carbohydrate loading, high myocardial uptake of F-18 FDG reflects increased myocardial glucose utilization due to the release of:
   A. Endogenous insulin
   B. Exogenous insulin
   C. Glucagon
   D. Pyruvate

129. Arrhythmias, such as multiple PVCs, can adversely affect the gated blood pool study if these beats account for more than:
   A. 5 %
   B. 10 %
   C. 20 %
   D. 30 %

130. In the Bruce protocol, the incline and speed of the treadmill are increased every 3 min through a total of:
   A. Five stages
   B. Six stages
   C. Seven stages
   D. Eight stages

131. To minimize hepatobiliary and gastrointestinal interference, the optimal time imaging window for Tc-99m-labeled radiopharmaceuticals (Sestamibi or Tetrofosmin) is:
   A. 10 min
   B. When radiotracer activity has cleared from the gastrointestinal tract and not concentrated in the liver
   C. When radiotracer activity has cleared from the liver and not concentrated in the gastrointestinal tract
   D. 30 min

132. The standard SPECT myocardial perfusion imaging projection views are
     acquired over:
     A. 90° arc
     B. 180° arc
     C. 270° arc
     D. 360° arc

133. Which of the following X-ray photons emitted from Tl-201 decay are primarily
     captured during imaging?
     A. 75–80 keV
     B. 135 keV
     C. 167 keV
     D. 135–167 keV

134. PET tracers: C-11 acetate and O_2-15 are markers of:
     A. Cell proliferation
     B. Glucose utilization and metabolism
     C. Membrane synthesis
     D. Oxidative and oxygen metabolism

135. Figure 2.4 presents a screenshot of a standard LAO view MUGA scan. The
     arrow is pointing to the:
     A. Left atrium
     B. Left ventricle
     C. Right atrium
     D. Right ventricle

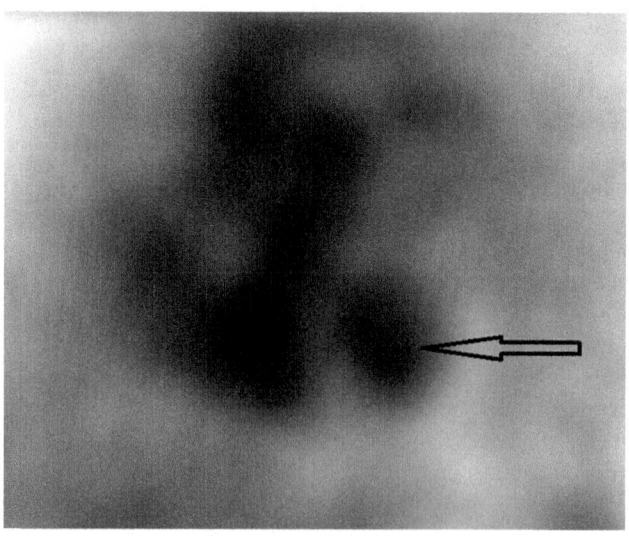

Fig. 2.4 Muga scan

136. Radiation exposure to patients from cardiac dual-isotope imaging (thallium and technetium) is approximately:
    A. 4–6 mSV
    B. 8–10 mSV
    C. 18–20 mSV
    D. 25–30 mSV

137. The recommended 5 ml (0.4 mg regadenoson) intravenous dose of Lexiscan should be administered:
    A. As an 1 min continuous peripheral intravenous infusion
    B. As a rapid (~10 s) injection
    C. As a slow (~30 s) injection
    D. As a 2-min continuous peripheral intravenous infusion

138. All patients undergoing MPI tests should receive a card documenting that they received a radioactive tracer for medical purposes. This card should include all of the following information EXCEPT:
    A. Facility name and location
    B. Patient diagnosis
    C. Patient first and last name
    D. The date of the test

139. In patients with a smaller heart, the ESV is underestimated more than the EDV, which can result in:
    A. No change to the LVEF
    B. An overestimation of the LVEF
    C. An overestimation or an underestimation of the LVEF
    D. An underestimation of the LVEF

140. Patients without flow limiting stenosis can increase myocardial blood flow during exercise by a factor of:
    A. 1–2
    B. 2–3
    C. 3–4
    D. 4–5

141. The main disadvantage of the dual-isotope simultaneous acquisition protocol is:
    A. Attenuation
    B. Downscatter
    C. Motion artifacts
    D. Study duration

142. During a gated blood pool acquisition, images of the heart are usually acquired in two or three standard projections. Which of the following views provide the best separation of the left and right ventricles?
     A. Anterior
     B. Right anterior oblique
     C. Left anterior oblique
     D. Left lateral

143. All of the following Tc-99m-based tracers have received U.S. Food and Drug Administration (FDA) approval for detection of CAD EXCEPT:
     A. Pyrophosphate
     B. Sestamibi
     C. Teboroxime
     D. Tetrofosmin

144. The advantages of PET myocardial perfusion imaging over SPECT include all of the following EXCEPT:
     A. Assessment of perfusion during treadmill exercise
     B. Higher spatial resolution
     C. Improved attenuation and scatter correction
     D. Potential for quantifying regional blood flow

145. The fundamental hypothesis of myocardial perfusion SPECT imaging is that the radiotracer is distributed in the myocardium:
     A. Directly proportional to the dose of radiotracer at the time of injection
     B. Directly proportional to the blood flow at the time of injection
     C. Inversely proportional to the blood flow at the time of injection
     D. Inversely proportional to the dose of radiotracer at the time of injection

146. Normal myocardial uptake of Tl-201 at stress indicates the presence of:
     A. Myocardial infarction
     B. Myocardial ischemia
     C. Viable myocardium
     D. Dysfunctional myocardium

147. Tomographic reconstruction of the heart projection images produces transaxial images called:
     A. Short-axis images
     B. Long-axis images
     C. Horizontal images
     D. Vertical images

148. A positron is a particle similar to an electron EXCEPT that it:
  A. Is heavier
  B. Has a positive electric charge
  C. Has no charge
  D. Is slower

149. Which of the following is NOT a recommended use of Tl-201 as a MPI tracer?
  A. Assessment of LV function
  B. Diagnostic assessment of CAD
  C. Prognostic assessment
  D. Viability assessment

150. Which of the following is the most reliable electrocardiographic marker of exercise-induced ischemia?
  A. T wave height decreased
  B. J point depression
  C. ST segment depression
  D. P wave height increased

151. MPI images acquired 2 h after initial injection of Tc-99m sestamibi represent a "snapshot" of blood flow conditions and tracer uptake at:
  A. The time of exercise beginning
  B. The time of injection
  C. The time of exercise ending
  D. The time of imaging

152. An infiltrated injection may compromise the MPI study by all of the following EXCEPT:
  A. Masking ischemia
  B. Producing poor quality images
  C. Altering distribution of the radiopharmaceutical
  D. Masking motion artifacts

153. Which of the following software packages is NOT employed in the measurement and analysis of left ventricle perfusion and function?
  A. Emory Cardiac Toolbox (ECT)
  B. Practice Management Software (PMS)
  C. 4D-MSPECT
  D. Quantitative Gated SPECT (QGS)

154. PET tracer F-18 FDG is a marker of:
  A. Cell proliferation
  B. Glucose utilization and metabolism
  C. Membrane synthesis
  D. Oxidative and oxygen metabolism

155. Figure 2.5 presents LV volume curve derived from an 8-frame gated myocar-
     dial perfusion study using 4D-MSPECT. Calculated EF of LV is
     approximately:
     A. 47 %
     B. 60 %
     C. 71 %
     D. 85 %

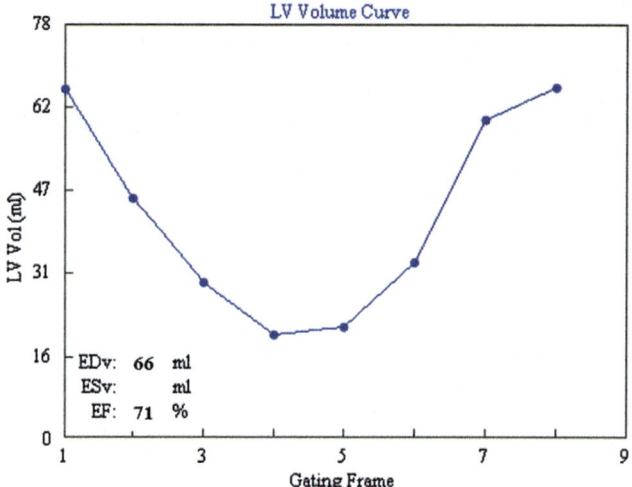

Fig. 2.5 Volume curve

156. The perfusion–metabolism match pattern—reduced perfusion and reduced
     metabolism—is indicative of:
     A. Hibernating myocardium
     B. Normal myocardium
     C. Scarred myocardium
     D. Stunned myocardium

157. The major pathway for excretion of Tc-99m sestamibi is the:
     A. Hepatobiliary system
     B. Skin
     C. Respiratory system
     D. Urinary tract

158. Tl-201 decays by electron capture to:
     A. Tl-202
     B. Tl-203
     C. Hg-201
     D. Hg-200

159. Patients undergoing tests with radionuclide administration should receive a card verifying that they collected a tracer dose of radioactivity for medical purposes. This card should include all of the following EXCEPT:
   A. The date of the test
   B. The referring physician name
   C. The location of the test facility
   D. The type of test

160. The resistance, against which the left ventricle must eject its volume of blood during contraction is called:
   A. Afterload
   B. Ejection fraction
   C. Preload
   D. Stroke volume

161. Which of the following views are obtained during the standard planar myocardial perfusion imaging acquisition?
   A. An anterior, a left lateral view, and a posterior view
   B. A left anterior oblique, a left lateral view, and a posterior view
   C. An anterior, a left anterior oblique, and a left lateral view
   D. A left lateral view, a posterior and right posterior oblique view

162. Labeling of red blood cells with Tc-99m pertechnetate requires stannous pyrophosphate which is:
   A. A buffer
   B. An oxidizing agent
   C. A reducing agent
   D. A stabilizer

163. Which of the following characteristics of Tl-201 limits its use in MPI SPECT imaging?
   A. High energy and short half life
   B. High energy and long half life
   C. Low energy and short half life
   D. Low energy and long half life

164. Which of the following positron emitting tracers is most frequently used to assess myocardial viability?
   A. C-11 acetate
   B. F-18 fluorodeoxyglucose
   C. N-13 ammonia
   D. Rb-82

165. The decision to temporarily stop medication prior to stress testing should always be done in consultation with the:
    A. Exercise physiologist
    B. Hospital pharmacist
    C. Referring physician
    D. Supervising physician

166. Which of the following imaging protocols provides information on both stress-inducible ischemia and viability?
    A. F-18 FDG viability imaging
    B. Tl-201 rest–redistribution imaging
    C. Tl-201 stress–redistribution–reinjection imaging
    D. Rb-82 perfusion imaging

167. Caffeine and methylxanthines limit the adenosine:
    A. Vasoconstricting effect
    B. Bronchodilating effect
    C. Vasodilating effect
    D. Positive chronotropic effect

168. Stunned or hibernating myocardium is:
    A. Dysfunctional and nonviable
    B. Nonfunctional but viable
    C. Dysfunctional but viable
    D. Nonfunctional and nonviable

169. Perfusion–metabolism mismatch—preserved metabolism in an area of decreased perfusion—is considered as the gold standard for:
    A. Myocardial infarction assessment
    B. Myocardial viability assessment
    C. Myocardial ischemia
    D. Myocardial arrhythmia

170. A 39-year-old woman presents to doctor's office with complaints of intermittent lightheadedness. She is asymptomatic and has no significant past medical, family, or social history. Her ECG (Fig. 2.6) shows:
    A. Atrial flutter
    B. Electronic ventricular pacemaker
    C. Normal sinus rhythm
    D. Sinus bradycardia

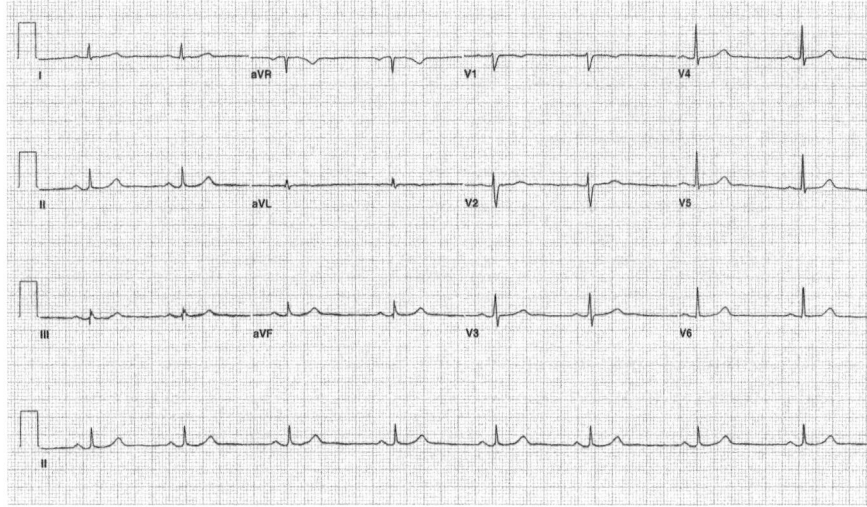

Fig. 2.6 Electrocardiogram

171. Which of the following gamma camera imaging techniques is DOSN'T assess ventricular function?
    A. Equilibrium gated radionuclide angiography
    B. First-pass radionuclide angiography
    C. Gated single photon emission computed tomography
    D. Infarct avid imaging study

172. All of the following types of muscular contraction or exercise can be applied as a stress to the cardiovascular system EXCEPT:
    A. Isobaric
    B. Isometric
    C. Isotonic
    D. Resistive

173. The major mechanism responsible for increasing coronary blood flow during stress involves a/an:
    A. Decrease in aortic diastolic pressure
    B. Increase in aortic systolic pressure
    C. Increase in coronary vascular resistance
    D. Reduction in coronary vascular resistance

174. The physical half-life of Rb-82 is:
    A. 38 s
    B. 58 s
    C. 78 s
    D. 98 s

175. Which of the following belongs do the right cardiovascular system (select three)?
    A. The left side of the heart
    B. The pulmonary arteries
    C. The pulmonary veins
    D. The right side of the heart
    E. The systemic arterial system
    F. The venous system

176. Which of the following factors/conditions can produce a false negative MPI study?
    A. Left bundle branch block
    B. Attenuation artifacts
    C. Patient motion
    D. Patient on calcium channel blockers

177. Tc-99m PYP has been used to image:
    A. Myocardial perfusion
    B. Myocardial necrosis
    C. Myocardial viability
    D. Ventricular function

178. The cardiac measurement defined as the blood volume pumped out by the ventricle over 1 min time period is called the:
    A. Ejection fraction
    B. End-diastolic volume
    C. End-systolic volume
    D. Cardiac output

179. Tc-99m-based MPI tracers are NOT recommended for:
    A. Assessment of LV function
    B. Diagnostic assessment of CAD
    C. Prognostic assessment
    D. Viability assessment

180. Absolute contraindications for exercise stress testing include all of the following EXCEPT:
    A. Acute pericarditis
    B. Decompensated congestive heart failure
    C. Electrolyte abnormalities
    D. Symptomatic cardiac arrhythmia

181. The most common computer-based methodology of global LV function assessment on GSPECT involves automated analysis of the:
    A. Apical and basal segments
    B. Epicardial and endocardial borders
    C. Apical segment and endocardial border
    D. Basal segment and epicardial border

182. During pharmacologic stress, intravenous coronary arteriolar vasodilators can increase coronary blood flow up to:
    A. 1–2 times above the resting level
    B. 2–3 times above the resting level
    C. 3–4 times above the resting level
    D. 4–5 times above the resting level

183. The magnitude of potential improvement of global LV function after revascularization is determined by the extent of:
    A. Ischemia
    B. Viable dysfunctional myocardium
    C. Viable nonfunctional myocardium
    D. Scar tissue

184. The high kinetic energy of Rb-82 positrons, together with the ultra-short physical half-life, produces myocardial perfusion images of:
    A. Low count density and high spatial resolution
    B. Low count density and low spatial resolution
    C. High count density and low spatial resolution
    D. High count density and high spatial resolution

185. The percentage of patients with CAD with a positive test result compared with the total number of patients tested with CAD describes the test:
    A. Specificity
    B. Sensitivity
    C. Accuracy
    D. Reproducibility

186. Figure 2.7 displays the schematic drawing of the normal heart conduction system. The label A represents the:
    A. Atrioventricular node
    B. Left bundle branch
    C. Right bundle branch
    D. Sinoatrial node

Fig. 2.7 Conduction system

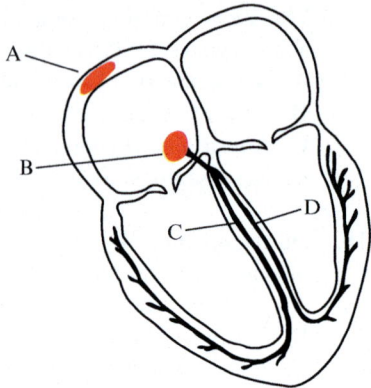

187. Which of the following medications can be used to attenuate severe and/or persistent adverse reactions to Lexiscan?
    A. Aggrenox
    B. Aminophylline
    C. Aspirin
    D. Atropine

188. The most common clinical manifestation of myocardial ischemia is:
    A. Angina pectoris
    B. Myocardial infarction
    C. Myocardial stunning
    D. Unstable angina

189. SPECT MPI is limited by the relative nature of the perfusion information; some patients with angiographically significant CAD may manifest a normal SPECT result because of:
    A. Balanced ischemia
    B. Irreversible ischemia
    C. Reversible ischemia
    D. Unbalanced ischemia

190. The double product units are:
    A. $mmHg \times beats/min \times 10^{-3}$
    B. $mmHg \times beats/h \times 10^{3}$
    C. $mmHg \times beats/h \times 10^{-3}$
    D. $mmHg \times beats/min \times 10^{3}$

191. On the morning of the day of testing, diabetic patients referred for a cardiac stress testing procedure should:
    A. Take their regular dose of insulin; do not eat a breakfast
    B. Take their regular dose of insulin; eat a light breakfast
    C. Not take insulin; eat a light breakfast
    D. Not take insulin; do not eat a breakfast

192. Which of the following MPI artifacts/findings can be resolved by performing delayed scanning?
  A. Apical thinning
  B. Diaphragm attenuation
  C. Liver attenuation
  D. Upward creep

193. During an ECG-gated SPECT acquisition, the "gate" opens when the peak of a/an:
  A. P wave is detected
  B. R wave is detected
  C. T wave is detected
  D. U wave is detected

194. The physical half-life of cyclotron produced N-13 ammonia is:
  A. 2 min
  B. 5 min
  C. 10 min
  D. 20 min

195. Reversible myocardial contractile dysfunction, in the presence of normal resting myocardial blood flow, is called:
  A. Myocardial infarction
  B. Myocardial ischemia
  C. Stunned myocardium
  D. Hibernating myocardium

196. In a typical gated SPECT acquisition, the first frame of the acquisition represents the:
  A. End-diastolic event
  B. End-systolic event
  C. Mid-diastolic event
  D. Mid-systolic event

197. Which of the following parts of Title 10 Code of Federal Regulations is concerned with the medical use of byproduct material, including the ALARA program, licensing, required surveys, instrumentation, and training requirements?
  A. 15
  B. 20
  C. 35
  D. 50

198. Visual comparison of a MPI stress and rest display revealing a perfusion defect that is seen on both the stress and rest images defines:
    A. A normal myocardium
    B. An ischemic myocardium
    C. A scarred myocardium
    D. A stunned myocardium

199. Tc-99m emits 140 keV of photon energy and has a physical half-life of:
    A. 4 h
    B. 5 h
    C. 6 h
    D. 7 h

200. Treadmill exercise ECG testing:
    A. Allows accurate localization of the site of myocardial ischemia
    B. Allows assessment of a patient functional capacity
    C. Allows measurement of left ventricle systolic function
    D. Allows accurate assessment of the extent of myocardial ischemia

201. The image presented in Fig. 2.8 was obtained during diagnostic cardiac:
    A. Computed tomography study
    B. Echocardiographic study
    C. Magnetic resonance imaging
    D. Myocardial perfusion imaging

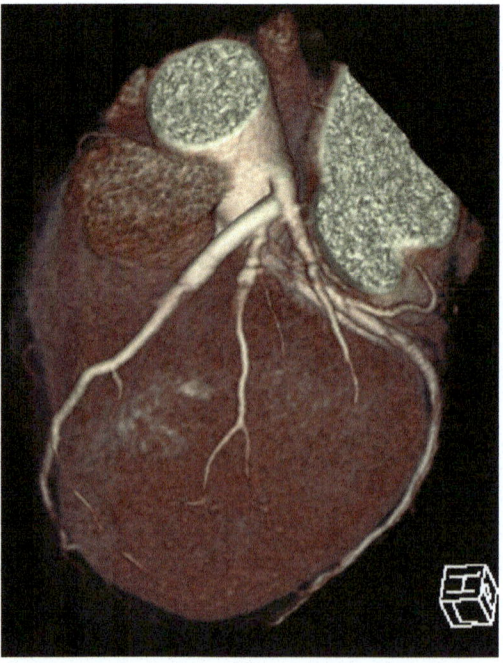

Fig. 2.8 Cardiac study

202. Which of the following is NO longer recognized in 10 CFR Part 20 and consequently is being phased out as an official unit for dose of record?
    A. Curie
    B. Rad
    C. Rem
    D. Roentgen

203. According to the NRC guidelines complete cessation of breastfeeding is suggested after administration of:
    A. Ga-67 citrate
    B. Tc-99m methylene diphosphonate
    C. Tc-99m pertechnetate
    D. Xe-133 gas

204. Fatty acids are:
    A. Amino acids
    B. Minerals
    C. Lipids
    D. Vitamins

205. The left main coronary artery (LM) derives from the left coronary sinus of Valsalva and gives origin to the left anterior descending coronary artery (LAD) and:
    A. The right coronary artery (RCA)
    B. The left circumflex coronary artery (LCX)
    C. The posterior descending artery (PDA
    D. The sinoatrial artery (SA)

206. Which of the following collimators is recommended for SPECT MPI?
    A. Low energy all purpose
    B. Low energy high resolution
    C. Low energy high sensitivity
    D. Medium energy

207. Patients referred for MPI study should avoid taking Viagra (sildenafil) before the study in the event that:
    A. Aminophylline is needed to counteract stress bronchospasm
    B. Nitroglycerine is needed to counteract stress-induced ischemia
    C. Propranolol is needed to counteract stress tachycardia
    D. Valium is needed to counteract stress-induced anxiety

208. Which of the following parameters from myocardial perfusion gated SPECT study DOESN'T describe diastolic function?
    A. Myocardial thickening
    B. Peak to filling rate
    C. Time to peak filling rate
    D. The mean filling fraction

209. Which of the following parameters describe the total of ischemic or jeopardized myocardium?
    A. Ejection Fraction (EF)
    B. Summed Stress Score (SSS)
    C. Summed Rest Score (SRS)
    D. Summed Difference Score (SDS)

210. The presented in Fig. 2.9 coronary angiogram shows:
    A. Normal coronary arteries
    B. 80 % occluded LM
    C. 80 % occluded LAD
    D. 80 % occluded LCX

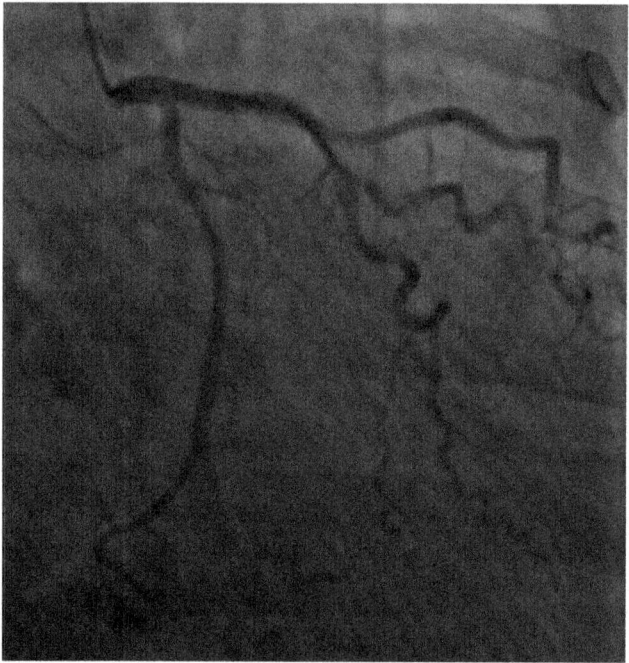

Fig. 2.9 Coronary angiogram

211. What area of myocardium is represented in the center of the SPECT MPI polar map?
    A. Apex
    B. Anterior wall
    C. Lateral wall
    D. Septum

212. Echocardiography use in standard chemotherapeutic monitoring of LV function is precluded by its:
    A. Availability
    B. Complexity
    C. Low specificity
    D. Low reproducibility

213. When the 2-day stress/rest protocol is employed, the stress study should be performed first because:
    A. The rest study can be omitted if the stress study is normal
    B. The stress study can be repeated if the rest study is normal
    C. There is no delay in reporting of the final analysis
    D. There is no need to alter patient medications

214. Which of the following SPECT MPI protocols offers the best image quality?
    A. 2-day stress/rest protocols
    B. Dual-isotope protocols
    C. Same-day rest/stress protocols
    D. Same-day stress/rest protocols

215. The image obtained during diagnostic cardiac angiography in Fig. 2.10 is called:
    A. Phase image
    B. Sinogram
    C. Spider view
    D. Ventriculogram

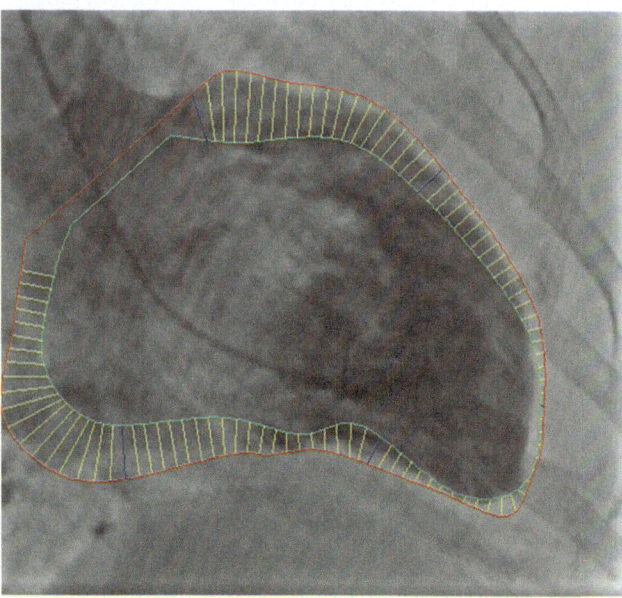

Fig. 2.10 Cardiac angiography

Answers

1. B. 85 %

   The first-pass myocardial extraction of Tl-201 is ∼ 85 %; however, only about 3–5 % of the total injected dose localizes in the myocardium when injected at peak exercise.
   (Zaret and Beller 2005)

2. D. Creates less liver and gut activity

   A well-known downside to technetium 99m-based imaging is the increased frequency of liver and gut activity in contrast to thallium-201.
   (Zaret and Beller 2005)

3. A. 0–4

   Perfusion is rated within each segment on a scale of 0–4, with 0 representing normal perfusion and 4 characterizing an extremely severe perfusion defect.
   (Bonow et al. 2011)

4. B. 124 s

   Measurements of myocardial blood flow necessitate close synchronization with the cyclotron O-15 production.
   (Schelbert 2009)

5. B. Coronary artery disease

   Atherogenesis is a process which leads to the formation of plaques made up of fatty materials. These plaques line the arteries, gradually constricting them. Inflammation plays an essential role in the pathobiology of a normal arterial wall becoming an atherosclerotic plaque.
   (Strauss et al. 2004)

6. D. Severe ischemia

   Ischemia-induced increase in left atrial and pulmonary pressures slows pulmonary transit of the tracer, allowing more time for removal or transudation into the interstitial spaces of the lung.
   (Dilsizian et al. 2009)

7. B. Dipyridamole

   Dipyridamole prevents intracellular reuptake and deamination of adenosine. The mechanism of inducing a perfusion abnormality is similar to that of adenosine, except true coronary steal occurs more frequently.
   (Iskandrian et al. 2003)

8. B. Oximetry

   Oximetry, performed noninvasively, can be employed to monitor arterial oxygen saturation, as long as a good signal pulse is obtained.
   (Jubran May 18 2012)

9. D. Thallium-201

   Peak myocardial concentration of thallium occurs within 5 min of injection, with rapid clearance from the intravascular compartment. The scintigraphic images obtained early after injection reflect the blood flow conditions at the time of tracer administration.
   (Bonow et al. 2011)

10. B. HR = 220 – age (in years)

    This formula tends to overestimate the maximum heart rate in the female population. A more accurate formula, offered in a study published in the journal, Medicine & Science in Sports & Exercise, is 206.9—(0.67 × age).
    (Bonow et al. 2011)

11. C. Infarction

    The summed stress score (SSS) characterizes the extent and severity of stress perfusion abnormality, the magnitude of perfusion defects related to both ischemia and infarction.
    (Bonow et al. 2011)

12. B. First-pass radionuclide angiography

    FPRNA is a useful technique for the measurement of the right ventricular (RV) function and quantification of a cardiac shunt.
    (Nichols et al. 1997)

13. B. Performing delay imaging

    The use of Tc-99m based agents with gated SPECT imaging is the well documented method of improving MPI specificity.
    (Bonow et al. 2011)

14. A. An electron

    A positron and an electron undergo mutual annihilation, and according to the law of conservation of energy, their masses are converted to 2 annihilation photons of energy, (gamma rays), each of energy about 511 Kev and moving in 2 opposite directions.
    (Lin and Alavi 2009)

15. A. stress-to-rest perfusion

    CFR provides a functional assessment of the severity of coronary stenosis—reduced CFR is seen in patients with hyperlipidemia; lowering cholesterol improves the CFR.
    (Yoshinaga et al. 2003)

16. C. diastolic blood pressure decreases

    In healthy patients during exercise, systolic blood pressure, mean arterial pressure, and pulse pressure usually increase. Diastolic blood pressure does not change considerably.
    (Bonow et al. 2011)

17. B. The ramp filter

    The Butterworth, Parzen, and Hamming are low pass filters that let low frequencies through. The Butterworth filters are the best of this group because the mathematical formula contains not only a cut-off frequency parameter but also the parameter called the order (roll-off).
    (Christian et al. 2004)

18. A. Avoid direct metal to skin contact

    The electrode fluid column can dry out over time with resulting poor-quality tracings.
    (Bonow et al. 2011)

19. C. extracardiac activity

    Extracardiac structure near the heart can produce counts that may reach the detector (falsely hotter cardiac region) or may cause a "ramp filter" or "negative lobe" artifact (falsely cold).
    (Bonow et al. 2011)

20. B. 3.5 ml O2/kg/min of body weight

    MET is useful to assess disability and standardize the reporting of submaximal and peak exercise workloads when different protocols are used.
    (Bonow et al. 2011)

21. B. Faster

    Thallium clearance is more rapid from normal myocardium with high thallium activity compared with myocardium with reduced thallium activity (differential washout).
    (Baggish and Boucher 2008)

22. B. Improving imaging characteristics

Adding exercise to vasodilator stress stimulates a blood flow to the skeletal musculature and away from intra-abdominal organs such as the liver. Low-level exercise is also an effective way of weakening vasodilator-related side effects.
(Thomas et al. 2000)

23. C. The summed difference score (SDS)

The summed difference score (SDS) is derived by subtracting the summed rest score (SRS) from the summed stress score (SSS).
(Bonow et al. 2011)

24. D. N-13 ammonia as a perfusion tracer and FDG as a metabolic marker of glucose use

A pattern FDG uptake in areas of hypoperfusion (described as "FDG/blood flow mismatch") suggests viable but hibernating myocardium.
(Lin and Alavi 2009)

25. A. Atheroma

The process that causes atheroma is termed atherosclerosis. Atheromas are confined within the wall of the vessel and typically occupy a fraction of the vessel circumference, and often extend from 1 to 2 cm.
(Strauss et al. 2004)

26. B. End-systolic

One of the frames in the middle of the acquisition (frame 4 in a typical gated SPECT acquisition where R-R interval is divided into eight frames) represents end-systolic events.
(Germano and Berman 2006)

27. C. Normal sinus rhythm

Common characteristics of sinus rhythms include: upright P waves that are similar in appearance, PR intervals of normal duration, and normal QRS complexes, provided that no ventricular abnormalities are present. By convention, normal sinus rhythm is usually defined as sinus rhythm with a heart rate between 60 and 100 beats/min.
(Goldberger 2006)

28. D. Viability study

Hibernation, and/or stress-induced ischemia demonstrated by SPECT imaging, is suggesting that this subpopulation of patients with heart failure may benefit from a noninvasive search for viability and ischemia.
(Cleland et al. 2003)

29. C. SPECT has shown a superior diagnostic performance when subanalyzed for gender

    PET overperforms SPECT when subanalyzed also for body mass index; the ability to identify multivessel ischemia with PET is significantly higher (74 % vs 41 %) than with SPECT perfusion imaging.
    (Bateman et al. 2006)

30. A. There are technical difficulties in monitoring systolic blood pressure

    A Gradual, reproducible decline in systolic blood pressure of 10 mmHg or more may indicate transient left ventricular dysfunction or an improper decrease in systemic vascular resistance, and is an indication to cease exercise if it is accompanied by other evidence of ischemia.
    (Bonow et al. 2011)

31. A. A bull's eye

    A polar map (bull's eye) representation—provides an overview of the entire three-dimensional myocardium in a two-dimensional plot.
    (Bonow et al. 2011)

32. D. Vascular space

    Ventricular cavity counts are used to generate a time–activity curve, from which functional parameters are derived.
    (Paul and Nabi 2004)

33. A. Additive to information from more available or less expensive tests

    Stress MPI data have been shown to have incremental prognostic value when added, for example, to clinical data information, stress ECG findings, and the Duke Treadmill Score.
    (Zaret and Beller 2005)

34. B. 1 month

    The physical half-life of Sr-82 is approximately 25 days. The generator can be eluted with >90 % yield every 10 min.
    (Takalkar et al. 2011)

35. B. A twofold to threefold

    Even though physical stress remains the preferred stress method for MPS, many patients are unable to exercise because of, e.g., arthritis, peripheral vascular disease, asthma, congestive heart failure, muscle diseases—for these patients, pharmacological stress is used as an alternative to physical exercise.
    (Iskandrian et al. 2003)

36. A. Dynamic exercise

Static exercise is isometric exercise that generates force with little muscle short-
ening that produces a greater blood pressure response than dynamic exercise.
(Williams et al. 2007)

37. C. 12 h

Ingestion of caffeine decreases the ability to detect reversible ischemic defect.
Products containing methylxanthines, including caffeinated coffee, tea, or
other caffeinated beverages, caffeine-containing drug products, and theophyl-
line should be avoided for at least 12 h before a scheduled radionuclide MPI.
(Astellas July 28 2012)

38. A. First-pass extraction fraction

With conventional SPECT imaging, the primary limitation is that the nonlinear relation of extracted tracer to myocardial blood flow imposed by lower
first-pass myocardial extraction causes a significant underestimation of exercise or vasodilator-induced increased blood flow and underestimation of flow
reduction caused by a flow-limiting stenosis.
(Bonow et al. 2011)

39. B. Is not adequately visualized

Outlining of the LV myocardium and LV cavity is achieved by delineating the
epicardial and endocardial borders on the perfusion image.
(Paul and Nabi 2004)

40. B. 64° and 72° F

Room temperature should be between 64° and 72° F (18° and 22° C) and
humidity should not exceed 60 %.
(Bonow et al. 2011)

41. B. Local myocardial perfusion

Simultaneously with washing out, thallium will be redelivered to the myocardium from a large reservoir in the blood pool— a region of ischemic but viable
myocardium which initially has less than normal uptake will become equal to
normal regions over time ("redistribution").
(Gibbons 2000)

42. D. 10 min after the exercise stress injection and 30–45 min after the pharmacological stress injection

Imaging is best done after a brief waiting period to allow for some liver and
biliary clearance, but before significant accumulation can occur in the transverse colon.
(Baggish and Boucher 2008)

43. B. slip ring technology

High-speed SPECT technology delivers true three-dimensional, patient-specific images localized to the heart. Compared with the traditional SPECT cameras, the high-speed SPECT systems can provide up to eightfold increase in count rates which results in reducing imaging times and radiation dose to patients.
(Erlandsson et al. 2009)

44. B. Hyperinsulinemic euglycemic clamp protocol

The utilization of the euglycemic hyperinsulinemic glucose clamp delivers excellent image quality, commonly displays uniform tracer uptake, and permits PET studies to be performed under steady and standardized metabolic conditions.
(Ghosh et al. 2010)

45. A. Infarcted myocardium

Patients with dysfunctional, but viable myocardium are likely to benefit from revascularization, whereas patients without viable myocardium will not benefit.
(Schinkel et al. 2007)

46. B. Ischemic myocardium

Myocardial ischemia progresses when coronary blood flow becomes insufficient to meet myocardial oxygen demand; myocardial cells switch from aerobic to anaerobic metabolism, with a gradual impairment of metabolic, mechanical, and electrical tasks.
(Bonow et al. 2011)

47. D. Sinus node dysfunction

Lexiscan can depress the SA and AV nodes and may cause first-, second-, or third-degree AV block or sinus bradycardia requiring intervention. Patients with implanted pacemaker scan undergo Lexiscan stress testing.
(Astellas July 28 2012)

48. C. Oil

The areas of electrode application are also rubbed with free sandpaper or a rough material to reduce skin resistance.
(Bonow et al. 2011)

49. C. 73 h

Tl-201 is generated in a cyclotron and must be delivered from a radiopharmacy.
(Early and Sodee 1995)

50. B. A treadmill speed of 1.7 mph and a grade of 10°

A standard maximal exercise treadmill protocol begins with a treadmill speed of 1.7 mph and a grade of 10° and increases both speed and grade every 3 min. (Bonow et al. 2011)

51. C. Delivers a higher radiation dose

The selection of radiotracer for MPI does not notably affect the distinction between the presence or absence of CAD. (Bonow et al. 2011)

52. C. R–R interval

Acquisition starts with the R wave on the ECG, which corresponds to the end diastole. The R wave to R wave interval (RR interval) is the inverse of the heart rate. (Paul and Nabi 2004)

53. C. McKesson Practice Choice Software

Methods of quantitative analysis of MPI have been developed to eliminate intraobserver and interobserver variability in the visual analysis of myocardial perfusion images. (Ficaro et al. 2012)

54. B. Energy of 3.15 MeV and average range of 2.8 mm

The physical characteristics of the positron emitted by Rb-82 are not completely optimal for imaging, resulting in somewhat impaired spatial resolution compared with F-18. (Takalkar et al. 2011)

55. C. 58 %

Ejection fraction (EF) represents the volumetric fraction of blood pumped out of the ventricle (heart) with each heart beat or cardiac cycle. Normal range 55–70 % (Schlosser et al. 2005)

56. B. At the onset of an ischemic response
C. Immediately after stopping exercise
F. The end of each stage of exercise
In the recovery phase the heart rate, blood pressure, and ECG should be recorded each minute for at least 5–10 min. (Bonow et al. 2011)

57. D. Second- or third-degree AV block

Adenosine should not be administered in patients with sinus node disease and second- or third-degree AV block (except in patients with a functioning artificial pacemaker).
(Astellas March 28 2012)

58. C. Doppler echocardiography

The advent of hybrid PET-CT has resulted in the unique opportunity to combine CT-derived morphologic information with PET-derived functional, physiologic, and biologic information.
(Heller et al. 2009)

59. A. End-diastole

Several dynamic images covering the length of the cardiac cycle—represented by the R–R interval—are acquired at equal intervals during an ECG-gated acquisition.
(Paul and Nabi 2004)

60. A. Accuracy

Accuracy can be calculated by using the formula: $(TP + TN/[TP + FP + TN + FN])$ where: TP-true positive, TN-true negative, FP-false positive, and FN-false negative.
(Koller 2002)

61. D. Patients with sinus rhythm

GSPECT should not be performed in patients with severe arrhythmia, such as atrial fibrillation, frequent premature ectopic beats, and heart block.
(Paul and Nabi 2004)

62. B. Tc-99m has a higher emission energy and a shorter half-life than Tl-201

Tc-99m has a higher emission energy and a shorter half-life than Tl-201, which permits administration of a higher dose with resulting improved image quality and contrast, and less soft tissue attenuation.
(Early and Sodee 1995)

63. C. Left bundle branch block

Breast and diaphragmatic attenuation, motion artifacts, processing errors, and cardiomyopathy can also result in false positive MPI.
(Zaret and Beller 2005)

64. B. Rb-82

Almost 21 years ago, the FDA approved Cardiogen-82 (Rubidium Rb-82 Generator) for MPI studies based on PET. Rb-82 has a short half-life (75 s), and is derived from strontium-82 (Sr-82), which has a half-life of 25 days. Rb-82 is collected from the generator column by injecting a solution of normal saline through the column.
(Heller et al. 2009)

65. B. ml O2/min per 100 g

Myocardial oxygen consumption is required to regenerate ATP that is utilized by membrane transport mechanisms and by myocyte contraction and relaxation.
(Klabunde July 21 2012)

66. D. Creates less liver and gut activity

A well-known downside to technetium 99m-based imaging is the increased frequency of liver and gut activity in contrast to thallium-201.
(Zaret and Beller 2005)

67. B. Flushing

The most common adverse reactions associated with adenosine infusion are flushing and chest discomfort. Adenosine is a potent peripheral vasodilator and can cause significant hypotension; however, patients with an intact baroreceptor reflex mechanism are able to maintain blood pressure and tissue perfusion by increasing heart rate and cardiac output.
(Astellas March 28 2012)

68. B. Anticoagulants

Heparin is a naturally occurring anticoagulant produced by basophils and mast cells and is not used orally; it is faster acting, as warfarin, given orally, usually takes a couple of days to reach the correct level.
(Kowalczyk and Donnett 1996)

69. A. adenosine, D. dipyridamole, E. regadenoson

Adenosine, regadenoson, and dipyridamole produce coronary vasodilation with resulting hyperemia. The detection of differences in coronary hyperemia between narrowed and normal vascular regions is the basis for production of perfusion defects by MPI.
(Zaret and Beller 2005)

70. A. Acute pulmonary embolism

Absolute contraindications for exercise stress testing also include uncontrolled hypertension and uncontrolled, symptomatic cardiac arrhythmias.
(Henzlova et al. 2010)

71. C. A moderate pretest likelihood of disease

    All diagnostic tests are of greatest value when there is an intermediate probability of disease, in the range of 50 %, and when the uncertainty is greatest.
    (Zaret and Beller 2005)

72. A. A 3-dimensional image volume can be reconstituted from a series of 2-dimensional images

    Tomographic reconstruction concept assumes that a 3-dimensional image volume can be reconstituted from a series of 2-dimensional images acquired at an adequate number of projections around the object being acquired, usually along an arc spanning at least 180°.
    (Germano 2001)

73. C. Allowing bed rest before SPECT

    Gravity has significant physiologic effects on the positions of organ systems, and a 5-min bed rest before SPECT acquisition appears to deliver enough time for the heart to adapt itself to its new position.
    (Karacalioglu et al. 2006)

74. C. Positron

    A positron rapidly annihilates with an electron, giving off two 511-keV photons, which travel in opposite (~1,800) directions.
    (Bengel et al. 2009)

75. A. The left side of the heart, C. The pulmonary veins, E. The systemic arterial system

    The right cardiovascular system comprises of the venous system returning deoxygenated blood to the heart, the right side of the heart, and the pulmonary arteries supplying blood to the lungs for gas exchange.
    (MacDonald and Burrell 2008)

76. A. The heart rate

    Calcium channel blocking drugs and beta-blocking drugs should be withheld on the day of diagnostic studies, though this should be done only if approved by the referring physician.
    (SNM May 28 2012)

77. A. Perpendicular to the long axis of the patient

    Transaxial is defined directed at right angles to the long axis of the body or a part.
    (Christian et al. 2004)

78. B. Two

One channel is open at both ends and permits urine to drain out into a collection bag. The other passage has a valve on the outside end and links to a balloon at the tip; the balloon is inflated with sterile water when it lies inside the bladder, in order to prevent it from sliding out.
(Kowalczyk and Donnett 1996)

79. A. 3 units lower

The 16-frame acquisition more precisely identifies the end systolic frame than the 8-frame acquisition.
(Germano et al. 1995)

80. A. Exercise

The MBF increases ~threefold with exercise, 2.5-fold with dobutamine, and three- to fivefold with vasodilator stressors.
(Iskandrian and Garcia 2012)

81. C. Upward creep

Upward creep of the heart during SPECT acquisitions may cause reconstruction artifacts and, therefore, false positive reversible defects.
(Karacalioglu et al. 2006)

82. A. Atrial fibrillation

AF is characterized by rapid, erratic electrical discharge that comes from multiple atrial ectopic foci. No organized atrial depolarizations are detectable. Atrial electrical activity on the ECG appears as irregular f (fibrillation) waves, varying continuously in amplitude, polarity, and frequency. Atrial fibrillation symptoms include heart palpitations, shortness of breath, and weakness.
(Goldberger 2006)

83. B. Kidneys

Intravenous administration of Tl 201 is characterized by rapid biexponential clearance from the blood, with about 91.5 % of blood radioactivity declining with a half-life of approximately 5 min, and the remainder with a half-life of about 40 h. Tl-201 is taken up by cardiac myocytes via the Na–K ATPase pump.

84. C. Pyruvate

The free energy released in this process is used to form the high-energy compounds ATP (adenosine triphosphate) and NADH (reduced nicotinamide adenine dinucleotide)
(Ghosh et al. 2010)

85. A. Specificity

    Sensitivity relates to the test's ability to identify positive results.
    Accuracy is the number of correct findings, regardless of whether the patient
    has CAD.
    (Munro 2005)

86. C. Coronary vasodilatation

    The production of cyclic AMP, stimulation of potassium channels, and
    decreased intracellular calcium uptake are responsible for coronary vasodila-
    tation induced by adenosine.
    (Heller et al. July 22 2011)

87. D. 10–20 s after the saline flush

    The radiotracer may be injected directly into the same catheter as Lexiscan.
    (Astellas July 28 2012)

88. B. Anticoagulants

    Anticoagulants, also referred to as blood-thinners, are used to stop platelets
    present in the blood plasma from clotting; they reduce risk for heart attack,
    stroke, and blockages in arteries and veins.
    (Kowalczyk and Donnett 1996)

89. C. The maximal 85 % of age-predicted heart rate is reached

    The currently used equation underestimates HR max in older adults and as a
    result underestimates the true level of physical stress imposed during exercise
    testing, and the fitting intensity of prescribed exercise programs.
    (Burrell and MacDonald 2006)

90. D. Symptoms

    In maximal (symptom-limited) stress testing, the patient continues to exercise
    at increasing levels until chest discomfort, significant hypertension or hypo-
    tension, gait problems, or severe dyspnea, etc. occurs.
    (Henzlova et al. 2010)

91. A. For every patient

    The attenuation correction map refers to automated techniques that accom-
    modate the intensity of the myocardial perfusion image to display the esti-
    mated degree of soft tissue attenuation on different regions of the heart and is
    patient specific.
    (O'Connor and Kemp 2006)

92. C. Is a nonspecific finding

Chest pain during vasodilator ST is a nonspecific finding because of involvement of adenosine A1 receptors in the nociceptive pathway influencing the sensation of chest pain.
(Udelson et al. 2004b)

93. C. Expensive

A numerical score is assigned to each of the groups—inappropriate 1–3, uncertain 4–6, appropriate 7–9, and the level of evidence is provided if available.
(Hendel et al. 2009)

94. A. Brightness

The common exemplification is the higher the number of counts the brighter the pixel.
In color images the relative differences in count values are represented by different colors.
(Iskandrian and Garcia 2012)

95. C. A L-R shunt

L-R develops because of the higher left-sided pressures; however, under chronic conditions right-sided heart pressures often increase, and may eventually even exceed left-sided pressures, producing a swap of flow and a R-L shunt.
(MacDonald and Burrell 2008)

96. D. Regadenoson

The recommended dose of Lexiscan is 0.4 mg regadenoson/5 ml administered by rapid intravenous injection and followed immediately by a saline flush and the radiopharmaceutical.
(Astellas March, 2012)

97. D. A

The end diastolic image is in frame # 1; the end systolic image is in frame # 16. A patient's LVEF and other quantitative information are obtained from the image that shows the best separation between the LV and RV, with visualization of the septal wall, which can usually be obtained with a left anterior oblique view. A minimum of 16 frames per R-R interval are required for an accurate assessment of ventricular wall motion and assessment of ejection fraction.
(Christian et al. 2004)

98. C. Chest compression

In the A-B-C sequence, chest compressions are often pushed back while the responder opens the airway to give mouth-to-mouth breaths, retrieves a barrier device, or collects and connects ventilation equipment.
(AHA May 25 2012)

99. B. The vasodilator stress agents

As adenosine has a very short half-life (~20–30 s), administration of aminophylline is rarely required during adenosine testing; simply stopping the infusion results in cessation of symptoms within 20–30 s.
(Ficaro et al. 2012)

100. C. Increases progressively to a peak response ranging from 160–200 mmHg

The higher range of the systolic blood pressure can be observed in older patients with more resistant vascular systems.
(Ellestad 2003)

101. C. Two-day protocol

The 2-day protocol is well suited to image obese patients and allows elimination of day 2 study if the stress study is normal.
(Husain 2007)

102. B. Short-axis view

The short-axis tomograms are displayed with the apical slices always shown first, then progressing serially toward the cardiac base. The left ventricle to the viewer's right and the right ventricle to the viewer's left. The superior surface is at the top and the inferior surface at the bottom.
(The Society of Nuclear Medicine July 1992)

103. C. How much does a test cost

The guidelines have been developed in the context of scientific data, the health environment, the patient's profile, and the physician's judgment.
(Hendel et al. 2009)

104. D. Rb-82

Cardiogen-82® (Rubidium Rb-82 Generator) contains accelerator produced strontium Sr-82 adsorbed on stannic oxide in a lead-shielded column and provides a means for obtaining sterile nonpyrogenic solutions of rubidium chloride Rb-82 injection.
(Rubidium Rb-82 Generator Sept 21 2012)

105. A. Within the first 10 day of the menstrual cycle

If, despite the patient being pregnant, the test cannot be postponed; particular attention should be provided to optimize the exposure to both the expectant mother and the unborn child.
(Grainger et al. 2001)

106. A. Increase in false positive studies

Attenuation artifacts are commonly revealed as a lasting perfusion defect that may incorrectly be accounted for as evidence of a coronary artery disease. Furthermore, these "defects" may display reversibility with changes in position and be confounded with myocardial ischemia.
(Zaret and Beller 2005)

107. B. 140 mcg/kg/min infused for 6 min

The recommended intravenous total dose of Adenoscan for adults is 0.84 mg/kg.
(Astellas March 28 2012)

108. A. Reduce the possibility of an infiltrated dose

If there is any uncertainty with respect to an infiltrated dose, a static image of the injection site should be acquired. The intravenous line used should be wiped clean afterward and disposed of properly.
(Burrell and MacDonald 2006)

109. D. Stress-induced echocardiographic changes

Completing the exercise stress in combination with MPI allows incorporating supplementary information on functional capacity, stress-induced electrocardiographic changes or arrhythmias, and use of heart rate reserve and heart rate recovery in the assessment of CAD probability or prognosis.
(Mark and Lauer 2003)

110. C. Old and frail

The modified Bruce protocol, which starts at a lower workload than the standard test, is typically used for exercise testing within 1 week of myocardial infarction, for elderly or sedentary patients, and for patients who are expected to have poor exercise tolerance for other reasons.
(MedicineNet.com May 10 2012)

111. D. Technetium first-pass myocardial extraction is 60 %; its energy results in less scatter and soft tissue attenuation

None of the clinically obtainable SPECT perfusion tracers have all of the properties of an ideal perfusion tracer; nevertheless, regional differences in myocardial tracer uptake during exercise or pharmacologic stress have provided important diagnostic as well as prognostic information.
(Ficaro et al. 2012)

112. C. Exercise

Dobutamine is a direct-acting inotropic agent whose primary activity results from stimulation of the ß receptors of the heart producing a dose-related increase in heart rate, blood pressure, and increased myocardial contractility.
(Dobutamine Feb 23 2012)

113. B. ± 10 % of the mean R–R interval

When the acceptance window is restricted, arrhythmic beats are rejected and the acquisition may be prolonged considerably.
(Paul and Nabi 2004)

114. C. O-15 water

Freely diffusible tracers accumulate and wash out from myocardial tissue as a function of blood flow, and they do not depend on a metabolic trapping mechanism.
(Bonow et al. 2011)

115. C. Radiation therapy

Morbidity and mortality due to MI can be reduced significantly if patients and witnesses recognize symptoms early, activate the EMS system, and in that way shorten the time to definitive treatment.
(Akinpelu October 11 2012)

116. A. ECFs on nuclear SPECT MPI are common and can be easily identified

Extracardiac incidental findings are observed in 1.7 % (0–2.8 %) of all cases, and 50 % of these are unsuspected prior to the study.
(Iskandrian and Garcia 2012)

117. B. Lexiscan, saline flash, radiotracer, saline flash

The myocardial perfusion imaging agent should be injected 10–20 s after the saline flush directly into the same catheter as Lexiscan.
(Astellas July 28 2012)

118. A. Hibernating myocardium

Higher degrees of mismatch have been shown to be associated with improved LV function with revascularization.
(Ghosh et al. 2010)

119. C. Injection

Because there is minimal redistribution of the radiopharmaceutical over time, imaging can be postponed and still provide accurate information about myocardial perfusion at the time of injection.
(Wheat and Currie 2005)

120. A. The double product

The double product is used as an indirect measure of myocardial oxygen demand—the peak rate-pressure product can be used to characterize cardiovascular performance.
(Bonow et al. 2011)

121. A. (EDV−ESV)/EDV × 100

The largest volume and the smallest volume represent the end-diastolic volume (EDV) and the end-systolic volume (ESV), respectively.
(Paul and Nabi 2004)

122. D. Transverse colon

A fatty meal may be used to speed hepatobiliary clearance of the sestamibi; however, there can be intense activity in the colon later, especially in patients with a high splenic flexure.
(Baggish and Boucher 2008)

123. B. 60 %

Myocardial uptake and clearance kinetics of both tracers are similar.
(Baggish and Boucher 2008)

124. A. F-18 FDG-6-phosphate

The 2' hydroxyl group (—OH) in normal glucose is needed for further glycolysis. F-18FDG is missing 2' hydroxyl and consequently FDG cannot be further metabolized in cells.
(Ghosh et al. 2010)

125. B. 70 ml

Stroke volume (SV) is the volume of blood pumped from one ventricle of the heart with each beat-normal range 55–100 ml.
(Schlosser et al. 2005)

126. D. Reinjection

After Tl-201 reinjection, approximately 50 % of regions with fixed defects on stress-redistribution imaging show significant enhancement of the tracer uptake, suggestive of improvement in regional LV function.
(Udelson et al. 2004a)

127. C. 5 ml (0.4 mg regadenoson)

Lexiscan is supplied in a single-use prefilled syringe: Injection solution containing regadenoson 0.4 mg/5 ml (0.08 mg/ml).
(Astellas July 28 2012)

128. A. Endogenous insulin

Released endogenous insulin also inhibits free fatty acids release from adipocytes leading to reduced circulating FFA.
(Fallavollita et al. 2010)

129. B. 10 %

In patients with atrial fibrillation, there may be considerable beat-to-beat variability, and the mean EF obtained during the period of acquisition may underestimate the actual LVEF.
(Dilsizian et al. 2009)

130. C. Seven stages

The protocol has seven stages, each taking 3 min, resulting in 21 min' exercise for a complete test.
(Hill and Timmis June 12 2012)

131. C. When radiotracer activity has cleared from the liver and not concentrated in the gastrointestinal tract

If there is a significant splanchnic or bowel overlap with the inferior wall, drinking water or milk or eating fatty food should be tried before repeating delayed imaging.
(Zaret and Beller 2005)

132. B. 180° arc

Projection views opposite the heart, i.e., LPO through RAO, spot considerably less myocardial activity due to attenuation through the patient's chest; those views provide mostly noise and scatter to the reconstruction, degrading overall resolution and contrast.
(Eisner et al. 1986)

133. A. 75–80 keV

The electron capture decay of thallium produces 88 photons at 70 to 80 keV and approximately 12 gamma photons at 135 and 167 keV for each 100 disintegrations. In spite of the excellent myocardial extraction and flow kinetic properties of thallium, its energy spectrum of 75–80 keV is suboptimal for conventional gamma cameras (ideal photopeak in the 140-keV range).
(Baggish and Boucher 2008)

134. D. Oxidative and oxygen metabolism

The cardiac muscle has a large number of mitochondria, enabling continuous aerobic respiration via oxidative phosphorylation, numerous myoglobins (oxygen-storing pigment), and a good blood supply, which provides nutrients and oxygen.
(Ghosh et al. 2010)

135. B. Left ventricle

The angle of the LAO projection is modified to obtain the best possible separation of the left and right ventricle. Tilting the detector head caudally will help separate the left ventricle from the left atrium.
(Christian et al. 2004).

136. D. 25–30 mSV

The American Society of Nuclear Cardiology strongly discourages use of dual isotope imaging on a routine basis with the exception of the assessment of myocardial viability.
(Cerqueira et al. 2010)

137. B. As a rapid (~10 s) injection

A 5 ml saline flush should be administered immediately after the injection of Lexiscan.
(Astellas July 28 2012)

138. B. Patient diagnosis

These patients may activate the alarms of the highly sensitive radiation detectors commonly used in public places, e.g., airports, government buildings, etc., by the Department of Homeland Security.
(Baggish and Boucher 2008)

139. B. An overestimation of the LVEF

An apparent shrinkage in the LV cavity observed in these patients is due to the partial-volume effect; zooming during the acquisition or reconstruction may reduce this error.
(Paul and Nabi 2004)

140. C. 3–4

The necessitated increase in blood flow must result from a decrease in vascular resistance, not through increase in blood pressure.
(Bonow et al. 2011)

141. B. Downscatter

The impact of scattered and primary photons from the first radionuclide into the photopeak window of the second radionuclide causes a significant degradation of image quality, image resolution, and quantitation errors.
(Henzlova et al. 2010)

142. C. Left anterior oblique

     Images of the heart are usually acquired in two or three standard projections: anterior, "best septal" left anterior oblique (best separation of the left and right ventricles) and optional left lateral (or left posterior oblique).
     (Zaret and Beller 2005)

143. A. Pyrophosphate

     Even though sestamibi, teboroxime, and tetrofosmin have received FDA approval, at present, only sestamibi and tetrofosmin are available for clinical use.
     (Baggish and Boucher 2008)

144. A. Assessment of perfusion during treadmill exercise

     The relatively short half-lives of both 82Rb-82 and N-13ammonia limit the utility of PET perfusion studies to patients undergoing pharmacologic stress only.
     (Bonow et al. 2011)

145. B. Directly proportional to the blood flow at the time of injection

     Generally, myocardial radiotracer uptake is linearly related to myocardial blood-under conditions of ischemia and mildly hyperemic flow; a linear relationship between myocardial perfusion radiotracer uptake and regional myocardial blood flow is preserved. At hyperemic flows, a relative decrease or "roll-off" in radiotracer extraction may be observed.
     (Iskandrian and Garcia 2012)

146. C. Viable myocardium

     Stress defects with redistribution (reversible defects) on 3- to 4-h delayed images is also a manifestation of viable myocardium.
     (Schinkel et al. 2007)

147. A. Short-axis images

     For the reason that the orientation of the heart relative to the patient's long axis differs from patient to patient, it has become a customary way to reorient the transaxial images into short-axis images.
     (Christian et al. 2004)

148. B. Has a positive electric charge

     The performance of positrons in tissue is very similar to beta particles; however, once a positron has been slowed down by atomic collisions, it is annihilated by interaction with an electron from a nearby atom.
     (Adam et al. 2008)

149. A. Assessment of LV function

Tl-201 has potential physical limitations for acquiring reliable ECG gated data, because the limited clinical dose and low energy compared with Tc-99m result in poor image quality, especially in ECG-gated images; the precision and accuracy of LVEF measurements with Tl-201 is debatable, particularly in cases of extended perfusion defects and poor count statistics.
(Baggish and Boucher 2008)

150. C. ST segment depression

The specificity of ST segment depression as the principal indicator of myocardial ischemia is limited. Decreased T waves, depressed J points and increased P waves are, among other, normal electrocardiographic changes observed during exercise.
(Banerjee et al. 2012)

151. B. The time of injection

As there is minimal clearance from the myocardium after initial uptake of this tracer, images acquired later than the initial injection represent a "snapshot" of blood flow and tracer uptake at the time of injection.
(Gibbons et al. 2000)

152. D. Masking motion artifacts

Since Tc-99m sestamibi, Tc-99m tetrofosmin, and Tl-201 can be picked up by tumors, visualization of lymph node activity on the cine raw data images ensuing from an infiltrated dose may mistakenly lead to an examination for malignancy.
(Williams et al. 2003)

153. B. Practice Management Software (PMS)

Direct comparison between these software packages showed excellent correlations in LV volumes and LVEF measurements.
(Nakajima et al. 2001)

154. B. Glucose utilization and metabolism

F-18 fluorodeoxyglucose has already set a standard in clinical care as a marker of glucose utilization in tissues exhibiting high glycolytic rates, including a broad spectrum of cancer types and ischemic but viable myocardium.
(Ghosh et al. 2010)

155. C. 71 %

Ejection fraction (%)=[ED (net)–ES (net)]÷ED × 100.
(Christian et al. 2004)

156. C. Scarred myocardium

The extent of scar has also been shown to be important in the prediction of LV function recovery after revascularization.
(Ghosh et al. 2010)

157. A. Hepatobiliary system

The high hepatic concentration may result in liver-dominant SPECT images with compromised cardiac resolution.
(Baggish and Boucher 2008)

158. C. Hg-201

Tl-201 has half-life of 73 h, emits Hg X-rays (~70–80 keV) and photons of 135 and 167 keV in 10 % total abundance. The lower-energy X-rays are captured during imaging.
(Baggish and Boucher 2008)

159. B. The referring physician name

For at least several hours after Tc-99m technetium-based MPI tracer injection and for a number of days after Tl-201 administration, patients may trigger the alarms of the highly sensitive radiation detectors now commonly used in public places.
(Baggish and Boucher 2008)

160. A. Afterload

Preload - the initial stretching of the cardiac myocytes prior to contraction- the end-diastolic volume (EDV) at the beginning of systole.
(Bonow et al. 2011)

161. C. An anterior, a left anterior oblique, and a left lateral view

The two-dimensional nature of planar imaging, in each of the standard views there is substantial overlap of myocardial regions; the tomographic (SPECT) perfusion imaging techniques replaced planar imaging as the standard acquisition and display methodology.
(Germano and Berman 2006)

162. C. A reducing agent

99m Technetium pertechnetate is bound to red blood cells using a variety of techniques. Three methods include the In Vivo Method, the Modified In Vivo/In Vitro Method, and the In Vitro Method.
(Saha 2004)

163. D. Low energy and long half-life

The long half-life requires lower doses to minimize risk of radiation exposure; the low energy leads to more image attenuation, especially in obese patients. (Baggish and Boucher 2008)

164. B. F-18 fluorodeoxyglucose

F-18FDG—a glucose analog in which one OH group is replaced by an F-18 atom—the initial tracer uptake in myocytes is comparable to glucose uptake. (Schinkel et al. 2007)

165. C. Referring physician

If the test is ordered for diagnostic purposes, beta-blocking and calcium-blocking medications, if possible, should be stopped 24 h before, or at the least on, the day of the procedure. Nitrates should not be taken on the day of the stress test.
(Zaret and Beller 2005)

166. C. Tl-201 stress–redistribution–reinjection imaging

The early uptake of Tl-201 largely depends on regional perfusion, while sustained uptake on cell membrane integrity (myocyte viability).
(Schinkel et al. 2007)

167. C. Vasodilating effect

Caffeine and methylxanthines block the adenosine receptors on arterial smooth muscle cells (A2b receptors) responsible for vasodilation in most vascular beds.
(Burrell and MacDonald 2006)

168. C. Dysfunctional but viable

Stunned or hibernating myocardium is dysfunctional but viable and has the potential to return to normal or improved contractile function with revascularization.
(Takalkar et al. 2011)

169. B. Myocardial viability assessment

Distinction of the viable myocardium from the nonviable myocardium before surgical intervention is imperative—dysfunctional but viable myocardium is potentially reversible and patients often benefit from surgery when quality of life and survival is considered.
(Zaret and Beller 2005)

170. D. Sinus bradycardia

Sinus bradycardia is a rhythm in which fewer than the normal—60–100 beats per minute—number of impulses arise from the sinoatrial (SA) node. Sinus bradycardia always needs to be interpreted in clinical context because it may be a normal variant or may be due to drug effect/toxicity, sinus node dysfunction, etc. Symptoms may include syncope, dizziness, lightheadedness, chest pain, shortness of breath.
(Goldberger 2006)

171. D. Infarct avid imaging study

Tc-99m-pyrophosphate myocardial scintigraphy does not provide information on the ventricular function; it is concentrated in the injured myocardium, primarily in areas of irreversibly damaged myocardial cells.
(Zaret and Beller 2005)

172. A. Isobaric

Isotonic exercise-dynamic or locomotory- primarily provides a volume load to the left ventricle. The cardiovascular response is proportional to the size of the muscle mass and the intensity of the exercise.
(Ellestad 2003)

173. D. Reduction in coronary vascular resistance

The major determinants of coronary blood flow include aortic diastolic pressure, which varies little during exercise, from the resting value, and a reduction in coronary vascular resistance, which is the major mechanism responsible for increasing coronary blood flow during stress.
(Bonow et al. 2011)

174. C.78 s

In spite of an ultrashort half-life, Rb-82 offers distinct logistical advantages. It is available through a generator that typically is operated by a semi-automated intravenous infusion system that makes possible close synchronization between pharmacologic or other stress interventions and the tracer administration.
(Schelbert 2009)

175. B. The pulmonary arteries, D. The right side of the heart, F. The venous system

The left cardiovascular system consists of the pulmonary veins returning oxygenated blood to the heart, the left side of the heart, and the systemic arterial system transporting blood to the body.
(MacDonald and Burrell 2008)

176. D. Patient on calcium channel blockers

Improper dietary/medication restrictions, e.g., caffeine consumption for pharmacologic stress studies, poor technique, and increased distance between patient and detector, can also result in false negative MPI.
(Zaret and Beller 2005)

177. B. myocardial necrosis

Tc-99m labeled pyrophosphate has been shown to bind to areas of necrosis and is believed to bind exposed mitochondrial calcium. (20 mCi min 4 h delay, within 12 h – 10 days post MI).
(Zaret and Beller 2005)

178. D. cardiac output

Cardiac output = Stroke Volume × Heart rate
An average resting cardiac output—5.6 L/min for a human male and 4.9 L/min for a female.
(Guyton and Hall 2006)

179. D. Viability assessment

There is minimal redistribution of these tracers compared with thallium.
(Baggish and Boucher 2008)

180. C. Electrolyte abnormalities

Acute myocarditis, poorly controlled congestive heart failure, and uncontrolled cardiac arrhythmias with hemodynamic compromise are also absolute contraindications for exercise stress.
(Henzlova et al. 2010)

181. B. Epicardial and endocardial borders

Multiple two-dimensional contours of the epicardial and endocardial borders of all of the tomograms in all three orthogonal planes are then reconstructed to create a surface-rendered three-dimensional display representing global LV function across a typical cardiac cycle.
(Germano and Berman 2006)

182. D. 4–5 times above the resting level

Myocardial regions supplied by stenotic coronary arteries have an attenuated hyperemic response. During exercise stress, coronary blood flow can increase approximately two to three times above resting levels.
(Bonow et al. 2011)

183. B. Viable dysfunctional myocardium

A dysfunctional territory with normal or only mildly reduced tracer uptake has a high likelihood of improved function after revascularization.
(Bonow 2002)

184. B. Low count density and low spatial resolution

Although myocardial perfusion images obtained with Rb-82 display lower count density and spatial resolution, the images are usually of good diagnostic quality.
(Schelbert 2009)

185. B. Sensitivity

Specificity relates to the ability of the test to identify negative results.
(Munro 2005)

186. D. Sinoatrial node

The SA node, a small mass of specialized cardiac tissue, is made up of Purkinje fibers, ganglion cells, and nerve fibers. It is located in the posterior wall of the right atrium of the heart that acts as a pacemaker by generating the electric impulses of the heartbeat at regular intervals.
(Bonow et al. 2011)

187. B. Aminophylline

Aminophylline may be administered in doses ranging from 50 mg to 250 mg by slow intravenous injection (50 mg to 100 mg over 30–60 s).
(Astellas July 28 2012)

188. A. Angina pectoris

Angina pectoris is caused by chemical and mechanical stimulation of sensory afferent nerve endings in the coronary vessels and myocardium and transmitted to the cerebral cortex.
(Alaeddini July 24 2012)

189. A. Balanced ischemia

Incorporation of other findings, including regional functional abnormalities from the gated portion of the examination, can be used to estimate more correctly the probability of disease and its extent.
(Dilsizian et al. 2009)

190. A. mm $Hg \times beats/min \times 10-3$

Most healthy individuals develop a peak rate pressure product of 20–35 $mmHg \times beats/min \times 10-3$.
(Bonow et al. 2011)

191. B. Take their regular dose of insulin; eat a light breakfast

Some labs advise patients, if they own a glucose monitor, to bring it with them to check their blood sugar levels before and after their exercise stress test.
(Diabetes and Stress Tests June 03 2012)

192. D. Upward creep

Delayed scanning time is also recommended in the presence of artifacts caused by increased liver activity (inferior or inferolateral defects are worse on resting images and with pharmacological agents).
(Karacalioglu 2006)

193. B. R wave is detected

ECG guides the acquisition so that the resulting set of SPECT images shows the heart as it contracts over the interval from one R wave to the next.
(Germano and Berman 2006)

194. C. 10 min

Because of the 10 min half-life, N-13 ammonia is logistically less demanding than oxygen-15–labeled (O-15) water that has a half-life of only 124 s.
(Schelbert 2009)

195. C. Stunned myocardium

Hibernating myocardium is ischemic myocardium supplied by a narrowed coronary artery, in which ischemic cells remain viable, but contraction is chronically depressed.
(Schinkel et al. 2007)

196. A. End-diastolic event

At a heart rate of 60 beats/min, each of the eight frames would comprise 125 ms—the first 125 ms after the peak of the initial R wave, and all imaging data that are recorded in frame 1 represent the end diastolic event.
(Germano and Berman 2006)

197. C. 35

NRC regulations that govern most nuclear medicine operations may be found in the CFR 10 parts 20, 30, and 35.
(Mettler and Guiberteau 2006)

198. C. A scarred myocardium

Myocardial scarring is fibrous tissue that replaces normal tissue destroyed by injury or disease pertaining to the muscular tissue of the heart, e.g., myocardial infarction, surgical repair of congenital heart disease.
(Ghosh et al. 2010)

199. C. 6 h

Tc-99m is eluted from molybdenum Mo-99 m in a generator and decays by isomeric transition with a physical T1/2 of 6.0 h.
(Early and Sodee 1995)

200. B. Allows assessment of patient functional capacity

Treadmill exercise ECG testing is widely available, inexpensive, and allows assessment of patient functional capacity. Imaging studies are indicated to localize the site or extent of myocardial ischemia and to assess myocardial viability.
(Weiner 2012)

201. A. Computed tomography study

3D volume rendered computed tomography (3D-CT) produces detailed, three-dimensional models that can be rotated and viewed in any orientation to provide a more natural and functional view of the patient's anatomy.
(Ropers et al. 2001)

202. D. Roentgen

Roentgen (R)—the dose of ionizing radiation that will produce 1 electrostatic unit of electricity in 1 cc of dry air—will still be seen on radiation survey instruments, and on radiation surveys, until the older models can be replaced. The radiation dose of record must be provided in rad or rem.
(NRC Accessed October 21 2012)

203. A. Ga-67 citrate

Only brief interruption (hours to days) of breast feeding is advised for Tc-99m macroaggregated albumin, Tc-99m pertechnetate, Tc-99m RBCs, 99mTc-WBCs, I-123 metaiodobenzylguanidine, and Tl-201.
(NRC Accessed Sept 1 2012)

204. B. Lipids

FAs are important component of lipids (fat-soluble components of living cells) in plants, animals, and microorganisms. Oleic acid, because it contains one double bond, is also denoted to as monounsaturated. Fatty acids that have multiple double bonds, e.g., linoleic acid are called polyunsaturated. Polyunsaturated fats are liquid at room temperature.
(Statkiewicz-Sherer et al. 2011)

205. B. The left circumflex coronary artery (LCX)

The LCX runs in the left atrial–ventricular sulcus and gives origin to obtuse marginal branches (OM), named from proximal to distal, OM1, OM2, OM3, and so on.
(Smuclovisky 2009)

206. B. Low energy high resolution

A high resolution collimator is recommended when imaging time can be extended and when good anatomical information is needed.
(Sharp et al. 2005)

207. B. Nitroglycerine is needed to counteract stress-induced ischemia

Nitroglycerine should not be given to a person who has recently taken Viagra, since the combination can cause a serious drop in blood pressure.
(Viagra Accessed Nov 23 2012)

208. A. Myocardial thickening

Parameters of diastolic function require a considerably greater number of gating intervals than are commonly exercised.
(Khalil 2011)

209. D. Summed Difference Score (SDS)

Summed Difference Score (SDS) is the difference between SSS and SRS.
(Fuster et al. 2007)

210. A. Normal coronary arteries

Similar to all planar angiograms, coronary angiograms are luminograms—one cannot see the wall of the vessel, only the contrast-filled lumen. Many times, it is difficult to grade a stenosis as having a single percentage value, and a range of percentage values is applied. Arteries that are totally occluded are referred to as total or 100 % occlusions.
(Ho and Reddy 2011)

211. A. Apex

The polar map represents the entire left ventricular volume, separated from the rest of the heart, with the tip of the apex turned toward the viewer in the center of the map.
(Zaret and Beller 2005)

212. D. Low reproducibility

Repeated analyses of the same ECHO recordings underestimate the clinically relevant interobserver reproducibility obtained by separate examinations by ~40 % for most measurements of LV function. Radionuclide gated equilibrium blood pool imaging provides rapid assessment with little discomfort but the high quantitative reproducibility.
(Ho and Reddy 2011)

213. A. The rest study can be omitted if the stress study is normal

The stress-rest sequence has theoretical advantages since a significant percentage of patients will have normal stress studies, thereby avoiding additional radiation exposure from a rest study.
(Ho and Reddy 2011)

214. A. 2-day stress/rest protocols

Two high doses on two separate days of Tc-99m labeled compounds produce the elevated high count rate, which enables high-quality images. The main disadvantage is the delay in reporting of the final analysis.
(Ho and Reddy 2011)

215. D. Ventriculogram

Left ventriculography is performed with coronary angiography, whereby a catheter is advanced into the left ventricle and contrast medium injected. Visualization of the left ventricle chamber allows assessment of the left ventricle function, e.g., measurement ejection fraction.
(Ho and Reddy 2011)

References and Suggested Readings

Adam A, Dixon KA, Grainger GR, Allison JD. Adam: Grainger & Allison's diagnostic radiology. 5th ed. St. Louis, MO: Churchill Livingstone; 2008.

AHA.   http://www.heart.org/idc/groups/heart-public/@wcm/@ecc/documents/downloadable/ucm_317350.pdf.

Akinpelu, D. ed. Treadmill stress testing. http://emedicine.medscape.com/article/1827089. Accessed 11 Oct 2012.

Alaeddini J. Angina pectoris. http://emedicine.medscape.com/article/150215-overview#a0104. Accessed 24 July 2012

Astellas. http://www.astellas.us/docs/.

Baggish LA, Boucher AC. Radiopharmaceutical agents for myocardial perfusion imaging. Circulation. 2008;118:1668–74.

Banerjee A, Newman DR, Van den Bruel A, Heneghan C. Diagnostic accuracy of exercise stress testing for coronary artery disease: a systematic review and meta-analysis of prospective studies. Int J Clin Pract. 2012;66(5):477–92.

Bateman TM, Heller GV, McGhie AI, et al. Diagnostic accuracy of rest/stress ECG-gated Rb-82 myocardial perfusion PET: comparison with ECG-gated Tc-99m sestamibi SPECT. J Nucl Cardiol. 2006;13:24–33.

Bengel MF, Higuchi T, et al. Cardiac positron emission tomography. J Am Coll Cardiol. 2009;54:1–15.

Bonow RO. Myocardial viability and prognosis in patients with ischemic left ventricular dysfunction. J Am Coll Cardiol. 2002;39:1159.

Bonow RO, Mann LD, Zipes PD, et al. Braunwald's heart disease – a textbook of cardiovascular medicine. 9th ed. Philadelphia, PA: Elsevier Saunders; 2011.

Burrell S, MacDonald A. Artifacts and pitfalls in myocardial perfusion imaging. J Nucl Med Technol. 2006;34:193–211.

Cerqueira MD, Allman KC, Ficaro EP, et al. Recommendations for reducing radiation exposure in myocardial perfusion imaging. J Nucl Cardiol. 2010;17:709.

Christian PE, Bernier DR, Langan JK. Nuclear medicine and PET: technology and techniques. 5th ed. St. Louis, MO: Mosby; 2004.

Cleland JG, Pennell DJ, Ray SG, et al. Myocardial viability as a determinant of the ejection fraction response to carvedilol in patients with heart failure (CHRISTMAS trial): randomised controlled trial. Lancet. 2003;362:14.

Diabetes and Stress Tests. http://diabetes.webmd.com/diagnosing-stress-tests? Accessed June 03 2012.

Dilsizian V, Narula J, Braunwald E, editors. Atlas of nuclear cardiology. 3rd ed. Philadelphia, PA: Current Medicine; 2009.

Dobutamine. http://www.drugs.com/pro/dobutamine.html

Early PJ, Sodee BD. Principles and practice of nuclear medicine. 2nd ed. St. Louis, MO: Mosby; 1995.

Eisner RL, Nowak DJ, Pettigrew R, et al. Fundamentals of 180 degree acquisition and reconstruction in SPECT imaging. J Nucl Med. 1986;27:1717–28.

Ellestad MH. Stress testing: principles and practice. 5th ed. New York: Oxford University Press; 2003.

Erlandsson K, Kacperski K, van Gramberg D, Hutton BF. Performance evaluation of D-SPECT: a novel SPECT system for nuclear cardiology. Phys Med Biol. 2009;54:2635.

Fallavollita JA, Luisi Jr AJ, Yun E, Dekemp RA, Canty Jr JM. An abbreviated hyperinsulinemic-euglycemic clamp results in similar myocardial glucose utilization in both diabetic and non-diabetic patients with ischemic cardiomyopathy. J Nucl Cardiol. 2010;17:637–45.

Ficaro EP, Hansen CL, American Society of Nuclear Cardiology: Imaging Guidelines for Nuclear Cardiology Procedures. Available at: http://www.asnc.org/imageuploads/ImagingGuidelines Complete070709.pdf. Accessed 22 May 2012.

Fuster V, O'Rourke RA, Walsh RA, Wilson P. Hurst's the heart. 12th ed. New York: McGraw Hill; 2007.

Germano G. Technical aspects of myocardial SPECT imaging. J Nucl Med. 2001;42:1499–507.

Germano G, Berman DS, editors. Clinical gated cardiac SPECT. Armonk, NY: Blackwell Futura; 2006.

Germano G, Kiat H, Kavanagh PB, et al. Automatic quantification of ejection fraction from gated myocardial perfusion SPECT. J Nucl Med. 1995;36(11):2130–47.

Ghosh N, Rimoldi EO, Beanlands SBR, et al. Assessment of myocardial ischaemia and viability: role of positron emission tomography. Eur Heart J. 2010;31:2984–95.

Gibbons JR. Imaging techniques. Myocardial perfusion imaging. Heart. 2000;83:355–60.

Gibbons RJ, Miller TD, Christian TF. Infarct size measured by single photon emission computed tomographic imaging with 99mTc-sestamibi: a measure of the efficacy of therapy in acute myocardial infarction. Circulation. 2000;101:101.

Goldberger LA. Clinical electrocardiography: a simplified approach. 7th ed. St Louis, MO: Mosby Elsevier; 2006.

Grainger GR, Allison JD, Adam A, Dixon KA. Grainger & Allison's diagnostic radiology: a textbook of medical imaging. 4th ed. London: Harcourt Publishers; 2001.

Guyton A, Hall EJ. Textbook of medical physiology. 11th ed. Philadelphia, PA: Elsevier; 2006.

Heller VG, Lundbye BJ, Kapetanopoulos A. Vasodilator stress radionuclide myocardial perfusion imaging: testing methodologies and safety. http://www.uptodate.com

Heller G, Calnon D, Dorbala S. Recent advances in cardiac PET and PET/CT myocardial perfusion imaging. J Nucl Cardiol. 2009;16(6):962–9.

Hendel CR, et al. ACCF/ASNC/ACR/AHA/ASE/SCCT/SCMR/SNM 2009 appropriate use criteria for cardiac radionuclide imaging. J Am Coll Cardiol. 2009;53(23):2201–29.

Henzlova JM, Cerqueira DM, Christopher L, HC H, et al. ASNC imaging guidelines for nuclear cardiology procedures. Stress protocols and tracers. J Nucl Cardiol. 2010;17:646–54.

Hill J, Timmis A. ABC of clinical electrocardiography. Exercise tolerance testing. http://www.ncbi.nlm.nih.gov/pmc/articles/PMC1123032/pdf/1084.pdf.

Ho BV, Reddy PG. Cardiovascular imaging. 1st ed. St Louis, MO: Saunders; 2011.

Husain SS. Myocardial perfusion imaging protocols: is there an ideal protocol? J Nucl Med Technol. 2007;35:3–9.

Iskandrian EA, Garcia VE. Atlas of nuclear cardiology: imaging companion to Braunwald's heart disease. Philadelphia, PA: Elsevier Saunders; 2012.

Iskandrian AE, Verani MS, et al. Nuclear cardiac imaging and principles applications. 3rd ed. New York: Oxford University Press; 2003.

Jubran A. Pulse oximetry. http://www.ncbi.nlm.nih.gov/pmc/articles/PMC137227/.

Karacalioglu OA, Jata B, Kilic S, et al. A physiologic approach to decreasing upward creep of the heart during myocardial perfusion imaging. J Nucl Med Technol. 2006;34:215–9.

Khalil MM, editor. Basic sciences of nuclear medicine. Berlin: Springer; 2011.

Klabunde ER. Cardiovascular physiology concepts. http://www.cvphysiology.com/CAD/CAD003.htm

Koller D. Assessing diagnostic performance in nuclear cardiology. J Nucl Cardiol. 2002;9:114–23.

Kowalczyk N, Donnett AK. Integrated patient care for the imaging professional. 1st ed. St. Louis, MO: Mosby; 1996.

Lin CE, Alavi A. PET and PET/CT. A clinical guide. 2nd ed. New York, NY: Thieme; 2009.

MacDonald A, Burrell AS. Infrequently performed studies in nuclear medicine: part 1. J Nucl Med Technol. 2008;36:132–43.

Mark DB, Lauer MS. Exercise capacity: the prognostic variable that doesn't get enough respect. Circulation. 2003;108:1534.

MedicineNet.com. Definition of Bruce protocol. http://www.medterms.com/script/main/art.asp?articlekey=30741

Mettler FA, Guiberteau MJ. Essentials of nuclear medicine imaging. 5th ed. Philadelphia, PA: Saunders Elsevier; 2006.

Munro HB. Statistical methods for health care research. 5th ed. Philadelphia, PA: Lippincott Williams & Wilkins; 2005.

Nakajima K, Higuchi T, Taki J, Kwano M, Tonami N. Accuracy of ventricular volume and ejection fraction measured by gated myocardial perfusion SPECT: comparison of 4 software programs. J Nucl Med. 2001;42:1571–8.

Nichols K, DePuey EG, Rozanski A. First-pass radionuclide angiocardiography with single-crystal gamma cameras. J Nucl Cardiol. 1997;4:61–73.

NRC. http://www.nrc.gov/reading-rm/basic-ref/teachers/05.pdf

O'Connor MK, Kemp BJ. Single-photon emission computed tomography/computed tomography: basic instrumentation and innovations. Semin Nucl Med. 2006;36:258266.

Paul KA, Nabi AH. Gated myocardial perfusion SPECT: basic principles. Technical aspects, and clinical applications. J Nucl Med Technol. 2004;32:179–87.

Ropers D, Moshage W, Daniel WG, Jessl J, Gottwik M, Achenbach S. Visualization of coronary artery anomalies and their anatomic course by contrast-enhanced electron beam tomography and three-dimensional reconstruction. Am J Cardiol. 2001;87:193–7.

Rubidium Rb-82 Generator. http://www.nuclearonline.org/PI/Cardiogen.pdf. Accessed Sept 21 2012.

Saha GB. Fundamentals of nuclear pharmacy. 5th ed. New York, NY: Springer; 2004.

Schelbert RH. Quantification of myocardial blood flow: what is the clinical role? Cardiol Clin. 2009;27:277–89.

Schinkel FLA, Poldermans D, Elhendy A, Bax JJ. Assessment of myocardial viability in patients with heart failure. J Nucl Med. 2007;48:1135–46.

Schlosser T, Pagonidis K, Herborn UC, et al. Assessment of left ventricular parameters using 16-MDCT: Results. Am J Roentgenol. 2005;184(3):765–73.

Sharp FP, Gemmell GH, Murray DA, editors. Practical nuclear medicine. 3rd ed. London: Springer; 2005.

Smuclovisky C. Coronary artery CTA. A case based atlas. Berlin: Springer; 2009.

SNM. Society of Nuclear Medicine Procedure Guideline for Myocardial Perfusion Imaging. http://interactive.snm.org/docs/pg_ch02_0403.pdf.

Statkiewicz-Sherer MA, Ritenour ER, Visconti PJ. Radiation protection in medical radiography. 6th ed. Maryland Heights, MO: Mosby; 2011.

Strauss WH, Grewal KR, Pandit-Taskar N. Molecular imaging in nuclear cardiology. Semin in Nucl Med. 2004;XXXIV(1):47–55.

Takalkar A, Agarwal A, Adams S, et al. Cardiac Assessment with PET. PET Clin. 2011;6: 313–26.

The Society of Nuclear Medicine, the American Heart Association, the American College of Cardiology. Standardization of cardiac tomographic imaging. J Nucl Med. 1992;33(7):1434–5.

Thomas GS, Prill NV, Majmundar H, Fabrizi RR, Thomas JJ, Hayashida C, et al. Treadmill exercise during adenosine infusion is safe, results in fever adverse reactions, and improves myocardial perfusion imagine quality. J Nucl Cardiol. 2000;7:439–46.

Udelson JE, Bonow RO, Dilsizian V. The historical and conceptual evolution of radionuclide assessment of myocardial viability. J Nucl Cardiol. 2004a;11:318.

Udelson JE, Heller GV, Wackers FJ, et al. A randomized, controlled dose-ranging study of the selective adenosine A2A receptor agonist binodenoson for pharmacologic stress as an adjunct to myocardial perfusion imaging. Circulation. 2004b;109:457.

Viagra. http://www.viagra.com/?source =google&HBX_PK=s_viagra&o=23121503|16637479310 &skwid=43100000390696855.

Weiner AD. Stress testing to determine prognosis and management of patients with known or suspected coronary heart disease. www.uptodate.com.

Wheat MJ, Currie MG. Rest versus Stress Ejection Fraction on Gated Myocardial Perfusion SPECT. J Nucl Med Technol. 2005;33:218–23.

Williams MA, Haskell WL, Ades P, et al. Resistance exercise in individuals with and without cardiovascular disease: 2007 update. A Scientific Statement from the American Heart Association Council on Clinical Cardiology and Council on Nutrition, Physical Activity, and Metabolism. Circulation. 2007;116:572.

Williams KA, Hill KA, Sheridan CM. Noncardiac findings on dual-isotope myocardial perfusion SPECT. J Nucl Cardiol. 2003;10:395–402.

Yoshinaga K, Katoh C, Noriyasu K, et al. Reduction of coronary flow reserve in areas with and without ischemia on stress perfusion imaging in patients with coronary artery disease: A study using oxygen 15-labeled water PET. J Nucl Cardiol. 2003;10:275–83.

Zaret BL, Beller GA. Clinical nuclear cardiology: state of the art and future directions. 3rd ed. Philadelphia, PA: Mosby; 2005.

Chapter 3
Practice Test #2: Difficulty Level—Moderate

Andrzej Moniuszko and B. Adrian Kesala

Questions

1. Peak myocardial concentration of thallium occurs within:
   A. 5 min of injection
   B. 10 min of injection
   C. 20 min of injection
   D. 40 min of injection

2. The most common configuration for cardiac transmission imaging uses a scanning line source of:
   A. Cobalt-57
   B. Gadolinium-153
   C. Cesium-137
   D. Technetium-99m

3. Which of the following protocols offers the potential of acquiring Tl-2011myocardial redistribution images?
   A. A single-day study low dose rest and high dose stress
   B. A 2-day study high dose rest and high dose stress
   C. A dual-isotope technique
   D. A single-day study high dose rest and low dose stress

Answers to Test #2 begin on page 120

A. Moniuszko, ARRT (N), PET, NCT. (✉) • B.A. Kesala, M.D.
Department of Radiology, Staff Radiologist, Presence Resurrection Medical Center,
7435 West Talcott Avenue, Chicago, Cook County, IL 60631, USA
e-mail: mdandy52@yahoo.com

A. Moniuszko and B.A. Kesala, *Nuclear Cardiology Study Guide: A Technologist's Review for Passing Specialty Certification Exams*, DOI 10.1007/978-1-4614-8645-9_3, © Springer Science+Business Media New York 2014

4. Which of the following statements correctly describes cardiac F-18 FDG uptake?
   A. Insulin inhibits cardiac F-18 FDG uptake; free fatty acids stimulate F-18 FDG accumulation
   B. Insulin and free fatty acids inhibit F-18 FDG accumulation
   C. Insulin stimulates cardiac F-18 FDG uptake; free fatty acids inhibit F-18 FDG accumulation
   D. Insulin and free fatty acids stimulate F-18 FDG accumulation

5. All of the following factors accelerate the process of the atheromatous plaque formation EXCEPT:
   A. Decreased high-density lipoprotein (HDL) cholesterol
   B. Increased levels of low-density lipoprotein (LDL) cholesterol
   C. Increased levels of homocysteine
   D. Decreased levels of homocysteine

6. A normal stress perfusion study is associated with a subsequent rate of cardiac death and myocardial infarction in less than:
   A. 1 %
   B. 5 %
   C. 10 %
   D. 15 %

7. Which of the following pharmacological stress agents assesses coronary flow reserve by increasing myocardial oxygen demand?
   A. Adenosine
   B. Dipyridamole
   C. Dobutamine
   D. Regadenoson

8. A 77-year-old female with a history of dyslipidemia and hyperthyroidism presents to the emergency department with heart palpitations, shortness of breath, and chest discomfort. Her ECG shows:
   A. Atrial fibrillation with rapid ventricular response
   B. Normal sinus rhythm
   C. Sinus rhythm with frequent PVC in a pattern of bigeminy
   D. Ventricular pacemaker

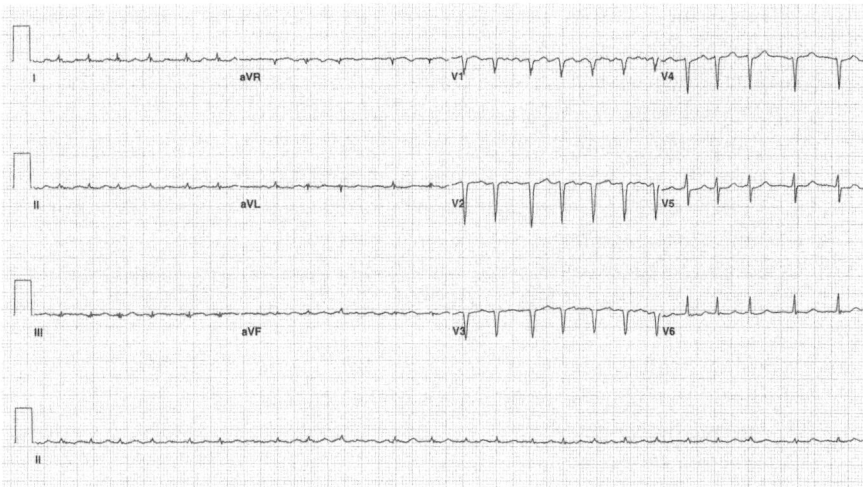

Fig. 3.1 Electrocardiogram

9. An imaging pattern in which the left ventricle or left ventricular (LV) cavity appears larger on the stress images than at rest is called:
   A. Cardiomegaly
   B. Cardiomyopathy
   C. Transient ischemic dilation
   D. Transient ischemic attack

10. At rest, the cardiac output and stroke volume:
    A. Are lower in a supine position than in an upright position
    B. Don't change with the position shift
    C. Are higher in a supine position than in an upright position
    D. Change in opposite directions with the position shift

11. Which of the following statements describing the concept of myocardial hibernation and/or stunning is FALSE?
    A. Myocardial hibernation and myocardial stunning may coexist in patients with ischemic cardiomyopathy
    B. Repeated ischemic attacks may induce repetitive stunning
    C. There is a temporal progression from stunning to hibernation
    D. There is a temporal progression from hibernation to stunning

12. Which view is recommended for performing a first-pass radionuclide angiography (FPRNA)?
    A. 20–30° LAO
    B. 30–50° LAO
    C. 30–50° RAO
    D. 20–30° RAO

13. Which of the following statements correctly describes lung uptake of Tl-201 and the Tc-99m-based tracers?
    A. Lung uptake may be missed with Tc-99m tracers because of the more delayed onset of imaging compared with thallium
    B. Lung uptake may be missed with Tl-201 because of the more delayed onset of imaging compared with Tc-99m-based tracers
    C. Lung uptake of Tl-201- and Tc-99m-based tracers is independent from the timing of imaging
    D. Lung uptake of Tc-99m-based tracers has been more extensively validated than lung uptake of the Tl-201

14. Which of the following PET algorithms uses the difference between arrivals of coincidence photons on both sides of the detector ring?
    A. Attenuation correction
    B. Random correction
    C. Scatter correction
    D. Time of flight

15. The physiologic process of programmed cell death, by which organisms selectively target cells to be eliminated when they are no longer needed, is called:
    A. Angiogenesis
    B. Apoptosis
    C. Arteriosclerosis
    D. Necrosis

16. In normal SPECT images, the lateral wall may often appear brighter than the contralateral septum because of:
    A. Structural variations of the myocardium—the apex is anatomically thinner than other myocardial regions
    B. Structural variations of the myocardium—the muscular septum is merging with the membranous septum
    C. Technical factors—the camera is physically farther away from the septal myocardial wall
    D. Technical factors—the patient motion

17. All of the following are the major vasodilators used for pharmacologic MPI EXCEPT:
    A. Adenosine
    B. Dipyridamole
    C. Dobutamine
    D. Regadenoson

18. Which of the following is identified as an index of the functional significance of a coronary stenosis?
    A. Coronary flow reserve (CFR)
    B. Myocardial blood flow (MBF)
    C. Summed rest score (SRS)
    D. Summed stress score (SSS)

19. The diaphragmatic attenuation artifact results in a perfusion defect in the myocardial segments commonly supplied by the:
    A. Right coronary artery territory
    B. Left coronary artery
    C. Left anterior descending artery
    D. Circumflex artery

20. During exercise, the value of arterial oxygen saturation normally does not decrease by more than:
    A. 1 %
    B. 5 %
    C. 10 %
    D. 20 %

21. If a point source and a 360°orbit are used, an alignment error between the center of the electronic matrix of the camera and the mechanical center-of-rotation (COR) is called:
    A. A bull's eye artifact
    B. A ring artifact
    C. A doughnut artifact
    D. A streak artifact

22. The primary reason that Tc-99m pyrophosphate has NOT gained widespread clinical use is its limitation in the detection of:
    A. Unstable angina
    B. Early infarction
    C. Viable myocardium
    D. Hypokinetic ventricle

23. Attenuation artifacts cause an increase in false-positive studies which results in MPI:
    A. Increased sensitivity
    B. Increased specificity
    C. Decreased sensitivity
    D. Decreased specificity

24. Which of the following tracers exhibits kinetic properties that very closely approach those of the ideal tracer of myocardial blood flow?
    A. Fluorine-18 (F-18) fluorodeoxyglucose
    B. Nitrogen-13 (N-13) ammonia
    C. Oxygen-15–labeled (O-15) water
    D. Rubidium-82 (Rb-82)

25. A state of persistent left ventricular dysfunction, resulting from a chronic and sustained reduction in myocardial blood flow is called:
    A. Myocardial infarction
    B. Myocardial ischemia
    C. Stunned myocardium
    D. Hibernating myocardium

26. If the position of the patient is different during stress and rest imaging, soft tissue attenuation artifacts may produce:
    A. An irreversible perfusion defect mimicking ischemia
    B. A reversible perfusion defect mimicking ischemia
    C. An elevated transient ischemic dilation
    D. Wall motion abnormalities

27. The application of three principles called justification, optimization, and limitation is aimed to:
    A. Restrict radiation dose
    B. Limit availability of diagnostic procedures
    C. Reduce availability of diagnostic radiopharmaceuticals
    D. Control employment

28. In patients with coronary artery disease, coronary flow reserve (CFR):
    A. Decreases in proportion to the degree of stenosis severity
    B. Increases in proportion to the degree of stenosis severity
    C. Increases in proportion to the level of exercise
    D. Decreases in proportion to the patient weight

29. The use of quantitative perfusion SPECT in myocardial perfusion imaging may assist in differentiating:
    A. Attenuation artifacts from true perfusion defects
    B. Horizontal from vertical motion artifacts
    C. Viable from necrotic myocardium
    D. Hibernating from stunning myocardium

30. Which of the following findings from exercise ST is least likely to be associated with an adverse prognosis and multivessel CAD?
    A. Early onset of angina
    B. Ischemic ST-segment depression
    C. Premature atrial contractions
    D. Fall in blood pressure at low exercise workloads

31. An increase in scintillator thickness will result in the camera's:
    A. Increased sensitivity and increased resolution
    B. Increased sensitivity and decreased resolution
    C. Decreased sensitivity and increased resolution
    D. Decreased sensitivity and decreased resolution

32. Which of the following medications will increase the sensitivity of Tc-99m-based tracers for detection of viable myocardium?
    A. Aminophylline
    B. Atropine
    C. Lasix
    D. Nitroglycerine

33. Electrocardiogram-gated SPECT offers useful:
    A. Anatomical information
    B. Epidemiological data
    C. Functional information
    D. Retrospective data

34. A PET study with which of the following tracers requires subtraction of blood pool activity?
    A. Fluorine-18 (F-18) fluorodeoxyglucose
    B. Nitrogen-13 (N-13) ammonia
    C. Oxygen-15–labeled (O-15) water
    D. Rubidium-82 (Rb-82)

35. Which of the following diagnostic modalities/procedures is considered the gold standard by which other diagnostic tests for CAD are judged?
    A. Echocardiography
    B. Electrocardiography
    C. Cardiac catheterization
    D. Cardiac computed tomography

36. Increased carbon dioxide production observed during exercise results in:
    A. Hyperthermia
    B. Hypertension
    C. Hyperventilation
    D. Hyperemia

37. Dipyridamole causes vasodilation:
    A. Indirectly by inhibiting reuptake of adenosine
    B. Directly by binding to adenosine type A2A receptors
    C. Indirectly by promoting reuptake of adenosine
    D. Directly by blocking adenosine type A2A receptors

38. Pattern of substrate uptake and utilization by the human myocardium in the fasting state is characterized by the:
    A. High rates of uptake and oxidation of glucose and lactate and the low rates of uptake of free fatty acid
    B. Low rates of uptake of glucose and lactate and the high rates of uptake and oxidation of free fatty acid
    C. Low rates of uptake of glucose and lactate and the low rates of uptake of free fatty acid
    D. High rates of uptake and oxidation of glucose and lactate and the high rates of uptake and oxidation of free fatty acid

39. The view comprising long-axis tomograms generated by slicing in the vertical plane through the short-axis perspective is called:
    A. Vertical short-axis view
    B. Horizontal short-axis view
    C. Vertical long-axis view
    D. Horizontal long-axis view

40. Automatic interpretations of ECG tracings are generally NOT accurate for:
    A. Cardiac axes
    B. Heart rates
    C. Intervals
    D. Repolarization abnormalities

41. Improving the spatial resolution of a collimator by restricting the range of incident angles will result in the collimator's:
    A. Decreased sensitivity
    B. Increased sensitivity
    C. Increased uniformity
    D. Decreased uniformity

42. Relative number of beats collected at a specific R-R intervals is called a beat:
    A. Electrocardiogram
    B. Histogram
    C. Sinogram
    D. Pictogram

43. The orientation that views the heart from the right ventricle to the left ventricle is called:
    A. Long-axis view
    B. Short-axis view
    C. Vertical long-axis view
    D. Horizontal long-axis view

44. Which of the following statements CORRECTLY describes the kinetic properties of Rb-82?
    A. Rb-82 displays a nonlinear relationship between blood flow and myocardial activity concentrations
    B. The first-pass extraction fraction of Rb-82 is higher than that of N-13 ammonia
    C. Rb-82, after intravenous administration, reaches the "plateau phase" at flows 3.0–3.5 mL/min/g
    D. The first-pass extraction fraction of Rb-82 is higher than that of oxygen-15–labeled (O-15) water

45. Flow through the coronary circulation depends on the pressure gradient between:
    A. The aorta and the left atrium
    B. The aorta and the right atrium
    C. The right and the left atrium
    D. The right and the left ventricle

46. The frequency at which the filter value is equal to 0.5 is called:
    A. Roll-off
    B. Cut-off
    C. Nyquist
    D. Fourier

47. All of the following pharmacological stress agents work directly on the coronary vessels to increase blood flow EXCEPT:
    A. Adenosine
    B. Dipyridamole
    C. Dobutamine
    D. Regadenoson

48. In healthy persons, the PR, QRS, and QT intervals:
    A. Shorten as heart rate increases
    B. Shorten as heart rate decreases
    C. Lengthen as heart rate increases
    D. Are independent from heart rate

49. The ability of the filters to both amplify and attenuate frequencies in selected ranges is a characteristic feature of:
    A. A low pass filter
    B. An active filter
    C. A high pass filter
    D. A ramp filter

50. Which of the following is the most common reason for stopping an exercise test?
    A. Arrhythmia
    B. Chest pain
    C. Fatigue
    D. Headache

51. Attenuation artifacts of the anterior and anterolateral myocardial walls may occur in men with:
    A. Anemia
    B. Cholelithiasis
    C. Gynecomastia
    D. Pneumonia

52. Which of the following frame times is recommended for a first-pass radionu-clide angiography (FPRNA)?
    A. 5 ms
    B. 25 ms
    C. 55 ms
    D. 85 ms

53. The Butterworth filter is an example of:
    A. A high pass filter
    B. A ramp filter
    C. An active filter
    D. A low pass filter

54. The images in a typical rest-stress myocardial perfusion study with Rb-82 chloride are acquired in the following order:
    A. Stress transmission scan, stress images, rest transmission scan, rest images
    B. Rest transmission scan, rest images, stress transmission scan, stress images
    C. Rest transmission scan, rest images, stress images, stress transmission scan
    D. Stress transmission scan, rest transmission scan, stress images, rest images

55. A 73-year-old man with a history of CABG, and with a family history of a younger brother who had coronary artery bypass surgery, presents to ED with complaints of intermittent lightheadedness and dizziness. His ECG (Fig. 3.2) indicates:
   A. Atrial flutter
   B. Normal sinus rhythm
   C. Sinus bradycardia
   D. Ventricular pacemaker

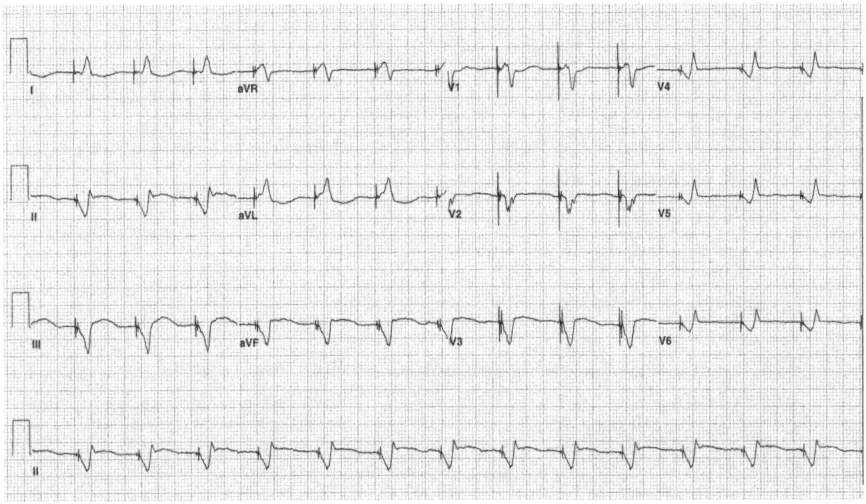

Fig. 3.2 Electrocardiogram

56. An exercise workload of 3–5 METs (metabolic equivalent of task) is consistent with:
   A. Standing
   B. Walking at 1–2 mph
   C. Walking at 3–4 mph
   D. Playing single tennis

57. An alkaloid that reduces vagal tone, consequently increasing the HR and enhancing conduction through the bundle of His is called:
   A. Aggrenox
   B. Aminophylline
   C. Aspirin
   D. Atropine

58. Which of the following is usually chosen as the isoelectric point for ECG interpretation?
    A. The beginning of the P wave
    B. The PQ junction
    C. the QR junction
    D. The ending of the T wave

59. Large, pendulous breasts are more likely to attenuate:
    A. The anterior myocardial wall
    B. The lateral myocardial wall
    C. The inferior myocardial wall
    D. The septal wall

60. Exercise myocardial perfusion studies in patients with LBBB mimic stress-induced ischemia in the:
    A. Apex
    B. Anterior wall
    C. Inferior wall
    D. Septum

61. Which of the following radiotracers has the shortest myocardial retention time?
    A. Tc-99m sestamibi
    B. Tc-99m teboroxime
    C. Tc-99m tetrofosmin
    D. Tl-201 thallous chloride

62. The radiotracer administration through an adenosine infusion line may result in:
    A. Atrial fibrillation
    B. Transient atrioventricular block
    C. Transient ischemia
    D. Transient tachycardia

63. Tc-99m tetrofosmin, when compared to Tc-99m sestamibi, has:
    A. A longer biological half-life
    B. More rapid liver clearance
    C. A longer physical half-life
    D. More rapid kidney clearance

64. Which of the following describes the positrons emitted by N-13 NH3?
    A. Energy of 1.19 MeV and an average range of 2.8 mm
    B. Energy of 3.15 MeV and an average range of 2.8 mm
    C. Energy of 3.15 MeV and an average range of 0.4 mm
    D. Energy of 1.19 MeV and an average range of 0.4 mm

65. An important cellular signaling molecule, as well as a powerful vasodilator with a short half-life of a few seconds in the blood, is called:
   A. Arginine
   B. Nitric oxide
   C. Nitrous oxide
   D. Nitroglycerine

66. Figure 3.3 represents the LV volume curve derived from an 8-frame gated myocardial perfusion imaging study using 4D-MSPECT. The end systolic volume (ESV) of the LV is approximately:
   A. 19 %
   B. 23 %
   C. 47 %
   D. 60 %

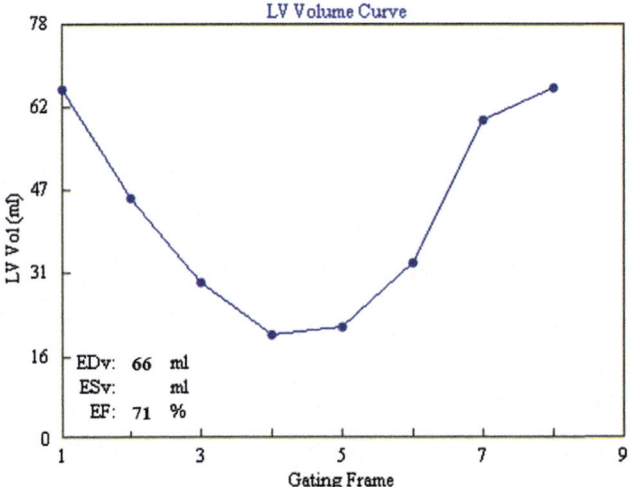

Fig. 3.3 Volume curve

67. Regadenoson stimulated coronary vasodilation and an increase in coronary blood flow (CBF) results from:
   A. Blocking of the A_{2A} adenosine receptor
   B. Inhibiting reuptake of adenosine
   C. Promoting reuptake of adenosine
   D. Triggering of the A_{2A} adenosine receptor

68. Myocardial oxygen consumption described as mixed venous oxygen saturation (MVO_2) at a resting heart rate is about:
   A. 2 ml O_2/min per 100g
   B. 4 ml O_2/min per 100g
   C. 8 ml O_2/min per 100g
   D. 16 ml O_2/min per 100g

69. Heterogeneity in myocardial blood flow (BF) in patients with CAD observed during a radionuclide stress test is caused by:
    A. Decreased BF in the normal territory and relatively unchanged BF in the territory supplied by the stenotic vessel
    B. Increased BF in the normal territory and relatively unchanged BF in the territory supplied by the stenotic vessel
    C. Increased BF in the normal territory and in the territory supplied by the stenotic vessel
    D. Decreased BF in the normal territory and in the territory supplied by the stenotic vessel

70. When estimating functional capacity, the amount of work performed should be measured in:
    A. The number of stages achieved
    B. Heart rate (HR)
    C. Metabolic equivalent (MET)
    D. The number of minutes of exercise

71. SPECT myocardial perfusion images usually use a standardized display in which data sets are normalized to:
    A. The maximum myocardial tracer content
    B. The mean myocardial tracer content
    C. The median myocardial tracer content
    D. The minimum myocardial tracer content

72. When equilibrium radionuclide angiocardiography (ERNA) is performed, the best septal view is usually achieved at:
    A. 150 RAO
    B. 45° RAO
    C. 15° LAO
    D. 45° LAO

73. Isolated reversible perfusion defect of the septum in patients with left bundle branch block (LBBB):
    A. Is commonly seen at low heart rates
    B. Is commonly seen in patients with low EF
    C. Is related to early relaxation of the septum
    D. Represents heterogeneity of flow between the LAD and left circumflex territories

74. PET camera electronics are created such that counts are recorded only when signals from opposite side detectors are registered:
    A. Within a timing window and along a line crossing COR
    B. Within a timing window and along a line of response
    C. Within an annihilation event window and along a line of response
    D. Within an annihilation event window and along a line crossing COR

75. Coronary artery disease (CAD) presents with a spectrum of diseases, from stable angina and unstable angina, to myocardial infarction. As per current guidelines, the particular syndrome is determined by all of the following EXCEPT:
    A. ECG findings
    B. Cardiac enzyme levels
    C. MPI findings
    D. Patient history

76. All of the following statements correctly describe advantages of single-isotope MPI over dual isotope imaging EXCEPT:
    A. Single-isotope MPI allows the opportunity to perform imaging with attenuation correction
    B. Interpretation of images is easier since the same isotope is used for both rest and stress
    C. TID markers can be determined much more easily with single isotope protocols
    D. Single-isotope MPI routinely evaluates myocardial viability

77. Figure 3.4 displays images acquired during a routine 32 frames multi-gated acquisition (MUGA) scan. The end systole image is labeled:
    A. D
    B. C
    C. B
    D. A

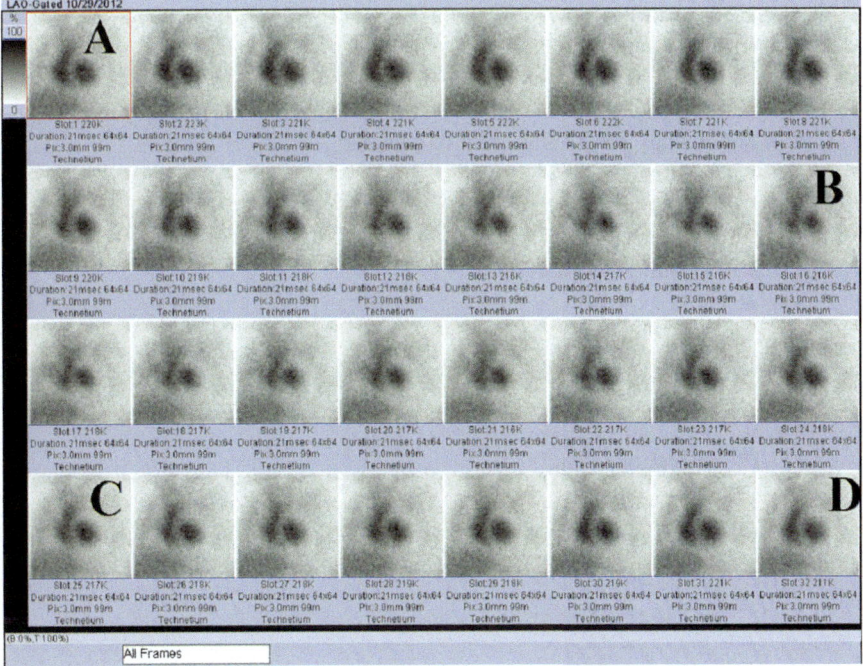

Fig. 3.4 MUGA scan

78. If the patient's resting heart rate is 60 beats/min, an 8-frame acquisition across the cardiac cycle comprises:
    A. 100 ms per frame
    B. 125 ms per frame
    C. 150 ms per frame
    D. 175 ms per frame

79. The presence of interventricular septal flattening on MPI SPECT studies indicates:
    A. Left atrial overload
    B. Right atrial overload
    C. Left ventricle overload
    D. Right ventricle overload

80. All of the following ECG changes observed during a stress test are classified as a positive ECG response to stress EXCEPT:
    A. ≥1 mm flat or downsloping ST depression 60–80 ms from the J point
    B. ≥1.5-mm upsloping ST depression 80 ms from the J point
    C. Premature atrial contraction
    D. ≥1-mm ST elevation

81. The appearance of the "Reverse redistribution" phenomenon can be created by all of the following EXCEPT:
    A. Tissue attenuation
    B. Motion artifact
    C. Dose extravasation
    D. Misalignment on SPECT slices

82. The administration of Tc-99m albumin aggregate particles when performing a R-L shunt study involves the risk of causing:
    A. A heart attack
    B. A microemboli in the brain
    C. Cardiac arrhythmia
    D. A macroemboli in the lungs

83. Sestamibi is principally cleared by:
    A. The hepatobiliary system
    B. Kidneys
    C. Skin
    D. The respiratory system

84. Voluntary motion of the patient in response to discomfort experienced in the course of PET/CT imaging most commonly occur:
   A. At the beginning of the scan
   B. During the CT study
   C. During the PET study
   D. During the acquisition of the topogram

85. Referral bias is a form of a systematic error that can result in:
   A. An overestimation of test specificity and an underestimation of test sensitivity
   B. An overestimation of test sensitivity and an underestimation of test specificity
   C. An overestimation of test sensitivity and test specificity
   D. An underestimation of test sensitivity and test specificity

86. Which of the following stress test modalities has the highest sensitivity for the diagnosis of CHD?
   A. Exercise ECG testing
   B. Positron emission tomography
   C. SPECT perfusion imaging
   D. Stress echocardiography

87. The maximal plasma concentration of regadenoson (Lexiscan) is achieved within:
   A. 1 min after injection of Lexiscan
   B. 1–4 min after injection of Lexiscan
   C. 4–8 min after injection of Lexiscan
   D. 8–12 min after injection of Lexiscan

88. The ventricle has two alternating functions-systolic ejection and:
   A. Asystolic relaxation
   B. Diastolic ejection
   C. Diastolic filling
   D. Systolic filling

89. Cadmium zinc telluride (CZT) crystals are:
   A. Solid-state detectors
   B. Liquid-state detectors
   C. Scintillation crystals
   D. Gas crystals

90. Which of the following exercise stress test findings/symptoms indicate a low probability of coronary artery disease (select three)?
    A. Chest pain
    B. Achieved 85 % of the maximum predicted heart rate
    C. Dyspnea at low work rate
    D. No ST segment depression
    E. A physiological response in blood pressure

91. Which of the following energy window settings is appropriate for the 70 keV and the 167-keV peak of Tl-201?
    A. 15 % and 15 %
    B. 15 % and 30 %
    C. 30 % and 15 %
    D. 30 % and 30 %

92. A vasodilator should be used in stress testing for patients unable to perform the standard exercise stress test or in patients who have (select two):
    A. Acute asthma
    B. Electronically paced rhythms
    C. Left bundle branch block
    D. Third-degree AV block
    E. Systolic blood pressure less than 90mmHg

93. False-negative (FN) test results of MPI relate to patients with:
    A. A positive test result who have CAD
    B. A negative test result who do not have CAD
    C. A positive test result who do not have CAD
    D. A negative test result who have CAD

94. The major inotropic/chronotropic agent used for pharmacologic radionuclide myocardial perfusion (rMPI) is:
    A. Adenosine
    B. Atropine
    C. Dipyridamole
    D. Dobutamine

95. A significant angiographic stenosis is present if a coronary artery is being narrowed by:
    A. 25 % or greater diameter reduction
    B. 45 % or greater diameter reduction
    C. 70 % or greater diameter reduction
    D. 90 % or greater diameter reduction

96. Figure 3.5 displays SA SPECT MPI images. Label D identifies the:
    A. Anterior wall
    B. Inferior wall
    C. Lateral wall
    D. Septal wall

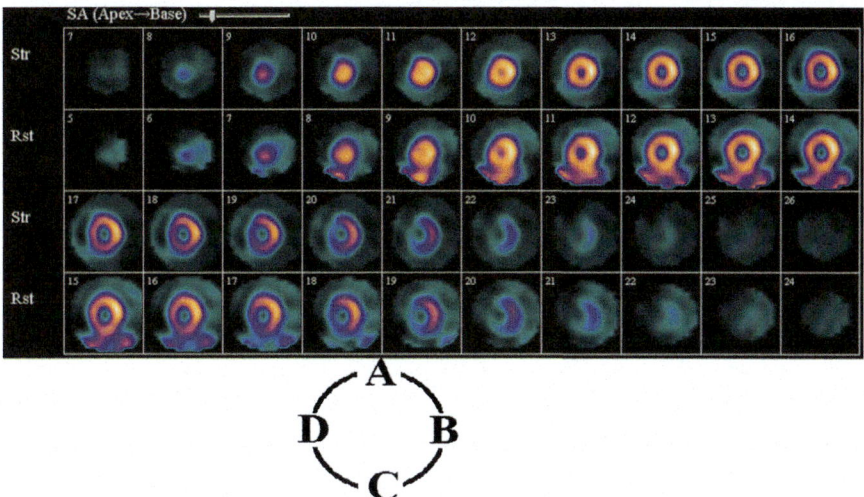

Fig. 3.5 SPECT MPI

97. Radiation exposure to patients from cardiac single isotope rest/stress technetium imaging is approximately:
    A. 4–6 mSV
    B. 8–10 mSV
    C. 18–20 mSV
    D. 25–30 mSV

98. The typical end-diastolic volume (EDV) for the left ventricle is approximately:
    A. 30 ml
    B. 60 ml
    C. 120 ml
    D. 240 ml

99. The American Society of Nuclear Cardiology (ASNC) recommends the use of stress-only imaging in all of the following groups of patients EXCEPT:
    A. Patients without known coronary artery disease
    B. Patients without known history of prior myocardial infarction
    C. Patients in the selected low or low-intermediate risk population
    D. Patients in the selected high-intermediate or high-risk population

100. All of the following are known confounders of exercise stress testing EXCEPT:
    A. Aggrenox
    B. Digoxin
    C. Left bundle branch block
    D. Left ventricular hypertrophy

101. Tl-201 decays by electron capture to:
    A. Ag-47
    B. Hg-201
    C. Tl-204
    D. U-235

102. Which of the following statements describing half-lives of the most widely available pharmacologic vasodilators is CORRECT?
    A. Regadenoson has a longer half-life than adenosine
    B. Adenosine has a longer half-life than dipyridamole
    C. Regadenoson has a longer half-life than dipyridamole
    D. Adenosine has a longer half-life than regadenoson

103. Which of the following groups of patients with suspected CAD have the highest rate of false-negative MPI tests?
    A. Patients with no disease
    B. Patients with low pretest probability of disease
    C. Patients with intermediate pretest probability of disease
    D. Patients with high pretest probability of disease

104. A PET acquisition, in which lead or tungsten septa divide detector rings such that only plane-by-plane LORs are detected, is known as:
    A. HD PET
    B. 2D PET
    C. 3D PET
    D. TOF PET

105. The difference between the amount of oxygen that enters the heart and that which leaves the heart per minute is called:
    A. The oxygen reserve of the heart
    B. The oxygen consumption of the heart
    C. The coronary blood flow
    D. The coronary flow reserve

106. The presence of a focal defect in rest images that was not seen on stress images, or a focal defect in stress images that appears more severe on rest images, is called:
    A. Reverse distribution
    B. Reverse redistribution
    C. Irreversible defect
    D. Reversible defect

107. Which of the following hemodynamic effects are the most common after administration of Lexiscan?
    A. A decrease in heart rate and in blood pressure
    B. An increase in heart rate and a decrease in blood pressure
    C. A decrease in heart rate and an increase in blood pressure
    D. An increase in heart rate and in blood pressure

108. Which of the following groups of patients have the highest risk of cardiac events when data from CT assessment of coronary-artery calcium (CAC) and information from MPI SPECT are combined?
    A. Patients with no CAC and normal SPECT MPI
    B. Patients with evidence of CAC and abnormal SPECT MPI
    C. Patients with evidence of CAC and normal SPECT MPI
    D. Patients with no CAC and abnormal SPECT MPI

109. A sestamibi kit for clinical use requires the addition of Tc-99m and must then be used:
    A. Immediately
    B. Within 6 h of preparation
    C. Within 12 h of preparation
    D. Within 24 h of preparation

110. Which of the following tests evaluating coronary artery disease is indicated in patients with an abnormal resting ECG?
    A. Exercise echocardiography
    B. Exercise stress test
    C. Treadmill MPI
    D. Planar imaging

111. Sensitivity and specificity of exercise and vasodilator stress myocardial perfusion SPECT with Tc-99m-based tracers for the detection of angiographically significant CAD is:
    A. 71 % and 91 %, respectively
    B. 89 % and 75 %, respectively
    C. 51 % and 79 %, respectively
    D. 91 % and 51 %, respectively

112. Which of the following radiopharmaceuticals is commonly used for detecting and quantifying R-L shunts?
    A. Tc-99m MAA
    B. Tc-99m MDP
    C. Tc-99m ECD
    D. Tc-99m DMSA

113. The reduction in intensity of a beam of gamma rays, due to absorption and scatter, is called:
    A. Absorption
    B. Adsorption
    C. Attenuation
    D. Addition

114. Adenosine is administered via an infusion pump at a dose of:
    A. 280 µg/kg per min for 6 min
    B. 140 µg/kg per min for 6 min
    C. 140 µg/kg per min for 8 min
    D. 2,800 µg/kg per min for 8 min

115. Which of the following is considered a risk factor for coronary artery disease?
    A. Cholesterol greater than 200 mg/dL
    B. Diastolic blood pressure greater than 90 mmHg
    C. Systolic blood pressure greater than 120 mmHg
    D. Sudden cardiac death in a first-degree relative younger than 75 years

116. Which of the following group of patients has the lowest ratio of non-diagnostic exercise stress test results?
    A. Patients with coronary artery disease
    B. Patients with orthopedic limitation
    C. Patients with peripheral vascular disease
    D. Patients with poor motivation

117. A 79-year-old woman presents with diabetes, breast cancer, progressive fatigue, anorexia, and several near-syncopal episodes. An ECG is performed in the office. Choose from the following responses to interpret this ECG (Fig. 3.6):
    A. Atrial flutter with rapid ventricular response
    B. Normal sinus rhythm
    C. Sinus rhythm with frequent PVC in a pattern of bigeminy
    D. Ventricular pacemaker

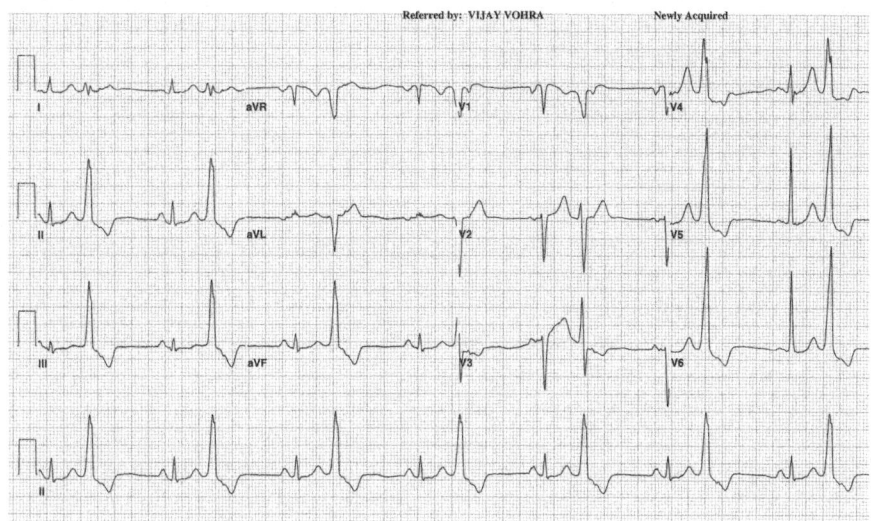

Fig. 3.6 Electrocardiogram

118. Which of the following statements describing risk stratification with coronary artery calcium (CAC) is FALSE?
    A. A high coronary calcium score indicates the presence of extensive calcification
    B. A high coronary calcium score is indicative of atherosclerosis
    C. A high coronary calcium score implies severe stress-induced perfusion abnormalities
    D. Stress SPECT MPI is an appropriate test to perform after CT imaging demonstration of CAC

119. What is the minimum amount of patient motion required to introduce a clinically significant artifact?
    A. Motion of 0.5 pixel
    B. Motion of 1 pixel
    C. Motion of 1.5 pixels
    D. Motion of 2 pixels

120. Failure to achieve a target age-predicted HR in the absence of positive ECG changes is regarded as:
    A. A negative test
    B. A non-diagnostic test
    C. A positive test
    D. An equivocal test

121. Methods that include either line source or computed tomographic (CT) techniques are employed to create:
    A. An emission scan
    B. An uniformity correction map
    C. An attenuation map
    D. A sinogram

122. All of the following are absolute contraindications for adenosine stress testing EXCEPT:
    A. Active bronchospasm
    B. Dipyridamole treatment
    C. More than first-degree heart block
    D. Systolic blood pressure more than 90 mmHg

123. Which of the following patients may require a second low dose of Tl-201 injection at rest to improve sensitivity for the detection of myocardial viability?
    A. Patients with arrhythmia
    B. Patients with hyperkinetic left ventricle
    C. Patients with severe hypertension
    D. Patients with severe ischemia

124. The most important advantage of PET imaging over SPECT is:
    A. Accessibility
    B. Less radiation exposure
    C. Increased sensitivity
    D. Increased specificity

125. A radiotracer injected into an arm vein that enters the coronary arteries circulates through (select correct order):
    A. The lung, the right atrium, the left ventricle
    B. The right ventricle, the right atrium, the lung
    C. The right atrium, the lung, the left atrium
    D. The right atrium, the lung, the left ventricle

126. The collimator–detector response (CDR) is determined by all of the following factors EXCEPT:
    A. Geometric response
    B. Intrinsic response
    C. Septal penetration
    D. Time of acquisition

127. The most common adverse reactions associated with regadenoson administra-
     tion are:
     A. Chest pain, nausea
     B. Flushing, abdominal discomfort
     C. Dyspnea, headache
     D. Feeling hot, dizziness

128. The most common cause of myocardial dysfunction in developed countries is:
     A. Alcoholic cardiomyopathy
     B. Diabetic cardiomyopathy
     C. Ischemic cardiomyopathy
     D. Obesity-associated cardiomyopathy

129. The magnitude of loss of spatial resolution is:
     A. Inversely proportional to the width and directly proportional to the length
        of the collimator hole
     B. Directly proportional to the width and to the length of the collimator hole
     C. Directly proportional to the width and inversely proportional to the length
        of the collimator hole
     D. Inversely proportional to the width and to the length of the collimator hole

130. Which of the following results of the Duke Treadmill Scores (DTS) identifies
     patient with moderate risk CAD?
     A. ≤ -11
     B. +4 to −10
     C. + 5 to + 10
     D. $\geq +10$

131. Segmentation, scaling, or a hybrid technique are used for:
     A. Scatter correction
     B. Motion correction
     C. Attenuation correction
     D. Randoms correction

132. In the LAO view, the orientation should be such that the long axis of the ven-
     tricle is approximately:
     A. Horizontal
     B. + 45°
     C. -45°
     D. Vertical

133. The administration of Tl-201 at peak stress must be performed in close proximity to the initiation of scanning, because delay in imaging will:
    A. Introduce motion artifacts
    B. Introduce attenuation artifacts
    C. Reduce image accuracy
    D. Reduce image quality

134. All of the following crystals are used in PET and PET/CT cameras EXCEPT:
    A. Gadolinium oxyorthosilicate
    B. Lutetium oxyorthosilicate doped with cerium
    C. Lutetium oxyorthosilicate doped yttrium
    D. Sodium iodide activated with thallium

135. A disorder characterized by progressive cardiac enlargement and contractile dysfunction is called:
    A. Dilated cardiomyopathy
    B. Myocardial infarction
    C. Stunned myocardium
    D. Restrictive cardiomyopathy

136. The property of a gamma camera that quantifies the size of the smallest object that can be determined reliably is called:
    A. Linearity
    B. Resolution
    C. Sensitivity
    D. Uniformity

137. Tomographic reconstruction of the heart projection images produces transaxial images which are:
    A. Perpendicular to the long axis of the patient
    B. Parallel to the long axis of the patient
    C. Perpendicular to the long axis of the left ventricle
    D. Parallel to the long axis of the left ventricle

138. The pattern of substrate uptake and utilization by the human myocardium in the fed state is characterized by the:
    A. High rates of uptake and oxidation of glucose and lactate and the low rates of uptake of free fatty acid
    B. Low rates of uptake of glucose and lactate and the high rates of uptake and oxidation of free fatty acid
    C. Low rates of uptake of glucose and lactate and the low rates of uptake of free fatty acid
    D. High rates of uptake and oxidation of glucose and lactate and the high rates of uptake and oxidation of free fatty acid

139. The myocardial distribution pattern of Tc-99m based tracers reflects:
    A. The myocardial perfusion at the time of acquisition and the LV function at the time of injection
    B. The myocardial perfusion at the time of injection and the LV function at the time of acquisition
    C. The myocardial perfusion and the LV function at the time of acquisition
    D. The myocardial perfusion and the LV function at the time of injection

140. In stage II of the Bruce protocol, the incline is adjusted to a 12 % grade and the speed is increased to
    A. 1.7 mph
    B. 2.5 mph
    C. 3.4 mph
    D. 4.2 mph

141. Which of the following SPECT segmentation models is recommended for the assessment of the myocardium and the left ventricular cavity?
    A. 15-segment model
    B. 17-segment model
    C. 20-segment model
    D. 24-segment model

142. The SPECT projection image consists of:
    A. A 2-dimensional snapshot of the 3-dimensional distribution of radioactivity
    B. A 3-dimensional snapshot of the 3-dimensional distribution of radioactivity
    C. A 3-dimensional snapshot of the 2-dimensional distribution of radioactivity
    D. A 2-dimensional snapshot of the 2-dimensional distribution of radioactivity

143. According to the AUC criteria, which of the following tests will be appropriate for evaluating a 54-year-old woman presented with atypical chest pain, hx of hypertension, hypercholesterolemia, and a normal resting ECG?
    A. Cardiac CT
    B. Coronary angiogram
    C. Exercise ECG
    D. Stress radionuclide MPI

144. PET tracers: C-11palmitate, F-18 fluoro-6-thia-heptadecanoic acid, and F-18-16-fluoro-4-thia-palmitate (FTP) are markers of:
    A. Cell proliferation
    B. Fatty acid metabolism
    C. Membrane synthesis
    D. Oxidative and oxygen metabolism

145. A ventricular septal defect (VSD) usually results in an L-R shunt because of the:
    A. Higher right than left ventricle pressure
    B. Higher right than left atrial pressure
    C. Higher left than right ventricle pressure
    D. Higher left than right atrial pressure

146. The major clinical consequence of soft tissue attenuation is that the resulting artifacts may be confused with:
    A. Foreign objects
    B. Extracardiac abnormalities
    C. True perfusion abnormalities
    D. Patient motion

147. The hemodynamic effect of adenosine is described as:
    A. A mild to moderate increase in mean BP associated with a reflex decrease in HR
    B. A mild to moderate increase in mean BP associated with a reflex increase in HR
    C. A mild to moderate reduction in mean BP associated with a reflex increase in HR
    D. A mild to moderate reduction in mean BP associated with a reflex decrease in HR

148. The reverse mismatch pattern—normal perfusion with relatively reduced metabolism—can be observed in patients with:
    A. Atrial fibrillation
    B. Chronic obstructive pulmonary disease
    C. Coronary artery disease
    D. Left bundle branch block

149. The variation in the length of the cardiac cycle during gSPECT may cause mixing of counts from adjacent frames with resulting:
    A. Attenuation artifact
    B. Motion artifact
    C. Spatial blurring
    D. Temporal blurring

150. The orientation that views the heart from the inferior surface looking toward the superior surface is called:
    A. Long-axis view
    B. Short-axis view
    C. Vertical long-axis view
    D. Horizontal long-axis view

151. Linear Energy Transfer (LET) is defined in units of:
    A. Kilovolt per micron
    B. Kilovolt per centimeter
    C. Kiloelectronvolt per micron
    D. Kiloelectronvolt per centimeter

152. All of the following are advantages of the first-pass technique over the equilibrium technique in cardiac imaging EXCEPT:
    A. High target-to-background ratio
    B. More distinct temporal separation of the cardiac chambers
    C. The potential for repeated assessment of cardiac function
    D. Quickness of imaging

153. Which of the following beats will be accepted in a patient with a heart rate of 72 beats per minute and if a 20 % acceptance window is used?
    A. Beats having duration of 0.66–0.88 s
    B. Beats having duration of 0.72–0.88 s
    C. Beats having duration of 0.72–0.96 s
    D. Beats having duration of 0.66–0.96 s

154. Temporal resolution in PET:
    A. Identifies radiotracer at low concentrations
    B. Allows photon attenuation
    C. Depicts tracer kinetics
    D. Corrects for scatter

155. The process of sprouting new capillaries from preexisting microvessels is called:
    A. Angiogenesis
    B. Apoptosis
    C. Arteriogenenesis
    D. Arteriosclerosis

156. All of the following are recognized absolute contraindications to exercise testing EXCEPT:
    A. Acute pericarditis
    B. Acute myocardial infarction (>2 days)
    C. Pulmonary embolism
    D. Uncontrolled hypertension

157. To image myocardial blood flow, SPECT perfusion tracers require the presence of myocyte viable:
    A. Sarcomeres
    B. Sarcoplasm
    C. Mitochondria
    D. Cell membranes

158. Figure 3.7 displays the schematic drawing of a normal heart conduction system. The label B represents the:
   A. Atrioventricular node
   B. Left bundle branch
   C. Right bundle branch
   D. Sinoatrial node

Fig. 3.7 Conduction system

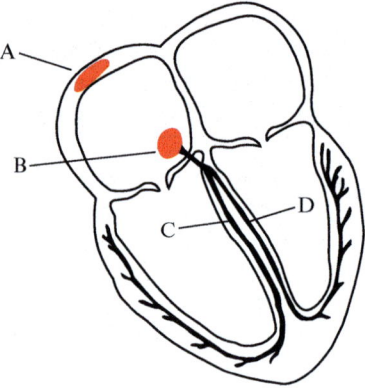

159. The ideal myocardial perfusion tracer should have all of the following qualities EXCEPT:
   A. Should be extracted rapidly
   B. Should be extracted completely
   C. Should be retained in myocardium
   D. Should be excreted via urinary tract

160. Which of the following medications should be withheld if the treadmill MPI study is being done for the primary diagnosis of coronary artery disease?
   A. Aggrenox
   B. Albuterol
   C. Aminophylline
   D. Nitroglycerine

161. According to the American Society of Nuclear Cardiology guidelines, immediate proceeding from rest to stress imaging during a 1-day protocol with Sestamibi or Tetrofosmin is acceptable as long as:
   A. The higher dose is 3.5–4.0 times the lower dose
   B. The higher dose is 2.0–3.5 times the lower dose
   C. The higher dose is 1.5–2.0 times the lower dose
   D. The doses are equal

162. Which of the following adenosine receptors mediate diminished heart rate and AV nodal conduction?
  A. A1
  B. A2a
  C. A2b
  D. A3

163. What is the main disadvantage of stress–rest protocols performed with Sestamibi or Tetrofosmin?
  A. Attenuation
  B. Degradation of image contrast
  C. Downscatter
  D. Longer study duration

164. Spatial resolution of current PET devices reaches…………. in the center of the field of view, compared with……… for SPECT:
  A. 8 mm, 10–12 mm
  B. 8 mm, 4 mm
  C. 4 mm, 4 mm
  D. 4 mm, 10–12 mm

165. Altered metabolic and contractile function that follows an ischemic episode is called:
  A. Hibernation
  B. Ischemia
  C. Infarction
  D. Stunning

166. The diagnostic accuracy of SPECT MPI to identify stenosis greater than 50 %:
  A. Is greater among men than among women
  B. Is greater among women than among men
  C. Is the same among women and men
  D. Is smaller in stenosis greater than 80 %

167. The damaging effect of radiation at high dose levels, such as those given in radiotherapy treatment, is an example of:
  A. Deterministic effect
  B. Fatal effect
  C. Fetal effect
  D. Stochastic effect

168. A phenomenon termed "posttest referral bias" is observed when:
  A. Patients with normal MPI are referred to coronary angiography
  B. Patients with abnormal MPI are referred to coronary angiography
  C. Patients with abnormal MPI are not referred to coronary angiography
  D. Patients with normal MPI are not referred to coronary angiography

169. The accuracy of gated single photon emission computed tomography (GSPECT) depends mainly on the proper delineation of the:
    A. Apex
    B. Base
    C. Endocardial contour
    D. Epicardial contour

170. An inappropriate increase in heart rate at low exercise workloads may occur in patients who are (select three):
    A. Bulimic
    B. Hypertonic
    C. Hypovolemic
    D. Overweight
    E. Physically deconditioned
    F. In atrial fibrillation

171. If a point source and an 180° orbit are used, an alignment error between the center of the electronic matrix of the camera and the mechanical center-of-rotation (COR) is called:
    A. Bull's eye artifact
    B. Ring artifact
    C. Tuning fork artifact
    D. Streak artifact

172. Which of the following radiopharmaceuticals is commonly used for detecting and quantifying R-L shunts?
    A. Tc-99m MAA
    B. Tc-99m MDP
    C. Tc-99m ECD
    D. Tc-99m DMSA

173. Figure 3.8 displays HLA SPECT MPI images. Label D identifies the:
    A. Apex
    B. Lateral wall
    C. Base
    D. Septal wall

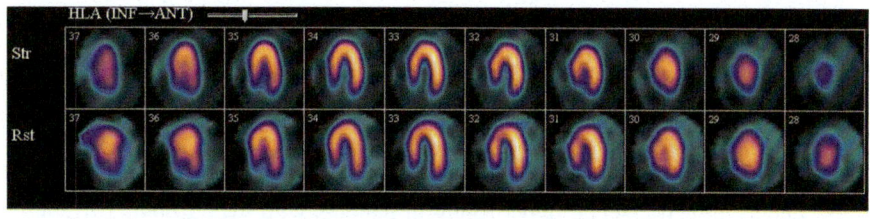

Fig. 3.8 SPECT MPI

174. Tc-99m diethylenetriaminepentaacetic acid (DTPA) is the recommended radionuclide of choice for first-pass RVG studies, because the DTPA:
    A. Is readily available
    B. Is cheap
    C. Enhances renal excretion
    D. Promotes Tc-99m RBC's binding

175. Radiolabeled vascular endothelial growth factor receptors (VEGFRs) have been targeted for imaging of:
    A. Angiogenesis
    B. Apoptosis
    C. Arteriosclerosis
    D. Atheromatosis

176. The inability to increase the heart rate to at least 85 % of age-predicted maximum is termed:
    A. Chronotropic incompetence
    B. Coronary insufficiency
    C. Inotropic incompetence
    D. Bathmotropic insufficiency

177. In-111 Antimyosin has been utilized for imaging of myocardial:
    A. Perfusion
    B. Necrosis
    C. Viability
    D. Function

178. In the USA, diseases of the heart and blood vessels are responsible for:
    A. ~20 % of all deaths
    B. ~ 40 % of all deaths
    C. ~60 % of all deaths
    D. ~ 80 % of all deaths

179. The asymmetric septal hypertrophy in patients with hypertrophic cardiomy-
    opathy (HCM) on polar map display can lead to the appearance of:
    A. A greater amount of tracer uptake in the inferior wall relative to the lateral wall
    B. A smaller amount of tracer uptake in the septum relative to the lateral wall
    C. A greater amount of tracer uptake in the septum relative to the lateral wall
    D. A smaller amount of tracer uptake in the inferior wall relative to the lateral wall

180. During strenuous exertion:
    A. Sympathetic discharge and parasympathetic stimulation are withdrawn
    B. Sympathetic discharge is maximal and parasympathetic stimulation is
       withdrawn
    C. Sympathetic discharge is withdrawn and parasympathetic stimulation is
       maximal
    D. Sympathetic discharge and parasympathetic stimulation are maximal

181. The greater hyperemic stress response achieved with vasodilator stress com-
    pared with an exercise stress test:
    A. Results in improved sensitivity to detect CAD
    B. Results in deteriorated sensitivity to detect CAD
    C. Has no effect on diagnostic accuracy
    D. Has not been evaluated

182. Reversal of the dipyridamole effect with infusion of aminophylline should be
    delayed, if it is clinically safe for at least 1–2 min after radionuclide adminis-
    tration because of:
    A. The antiarrhythmic effects would be reversed
    B. The coronary vasoconstricting effects would be reversed
    C. The coronary vasodilator effects would be reversed
    D. The inotropic effects would be reversed

183. The diagnostic ability of the pharmacologic stress test with dobutamine is
    limited because:
    A. Maximal heart rate is not achieved as often as with exercise stress
    B. Maximal coronary flow reserve is not achieved as often as with vasodilator
       pharmacologic stress
    C. Maximal heart rate is not achieved as often as with vasodilator pharmaco-
       logic stress
    D. Maximal coronary flow reserve is limited after atropine administration

184. To measure the PET attenuation correction factor, a rod that rotates about the patient is filled with relatively long-lived:
    A. Positron emitters germanium-68 or cesium-137
    B. Positron emitter germanium-68 or a single-photon emittercesium-137
    C. Positron emitter cesium-137 or a single-photon emittergermanium-68
    D. Single-photon emitters germanium-68 or cesium-137

185. Decreased cardiac output and sign of tissue hypoxia in the presence of adequate intravascular volume describe:
    A. Anaphylactic shock
    B. Cardiogenic shock
    C. Hypovolemic shock
    D. Septic shock

186. The degree of tracer uptake in hibernating or stunning myocardium directly reflects:
    A. The tracer dose
    B. The amount of preserved tissue
    C. The degree of dyskinesia
    D. The amount of scar tissue

187. The magnitude of the sinusoid in the Fourier sinusoidal image corresponds to its:
    A. Phase
    B. Contrast
    C. Frequency
    D. Resolution

188. The most common cause of heart failure in developed countries is:
    A. Alcoholic cardiomyopathy
    B. Chronic myocarditis
    C. Coronary artery disease
    D. Acute pericarditis

189. Which of the following groups of patients with suspected CAD will have a high rate of false-positive MPI tests?
    A. Patients with no disease
    B. Patients with low pretest probability of disease
    C. Patients with intermediate pretest probability of disease
    D. Patients with high pretest probability of disease

190. A composite index that was designed to provide survival estimates based on results from the exercise test, including ST-segment depression, chest pain, and exercise duration, is called:
    A. The angina index
    B. The Duke treadmill score
    C. Survival assessment
    D. Hard events predictor

191. On gated SPECT, during normal systolic wall thickening, it appears that the LV wall becomes:
    A. Brighter and thinner
    B. Darker and thicker
    C. Brighter and thicker
    D. Darker and thinner

192. All of the following frequently used drugs are known to interfere with red blood cell labeling EXCEPT:
    A. Digoxin
    B. Heparin
    C. Propranolol
    D. Valium

193. All of the following are advantages of planar imaging over SPECT imaging EXCEPT:
    A. Planar imaging doesn't require extensive image processing
    B. Planar imaging is less affected by patient motion
    C. Planar imaging has more ability to differentiate smaller perfusion abnormalities
    D. In planar imaging there are fewer sources of potential error and artifact

194. The proportion of coincident counts of a blank scan and a transmission scan generates the range of attenuation correction factors needed to correct each:
    A. Coincidence event
    B. Coincidence window
    C. Projection angle
    D. Projection line

195. The typical end-systolic volume (ESV) for the left ventricle is approximately:
    A. 25 ml
    B. 50 ml
    C. 100 ml
    D. 200 ml

196. Which of the following statements correctly describes a standard gSPECT acquisition and reconstruction?
   A. For perfusion analysis, raw data are reconstructed frame by frame
   B. For functional analysis, the frames are summed together
   C. Gated projection data require more smoothing than ungated data
   D. Errors during image acquisition will not compromise the accuracy of the measurements

197. False-positive (FP) test results of MPI refer to patients with:
   A. A positive test result who have CAD
   B. A negative test result who do not have CAD
   C. A positive test result who do not have CAD
   D. A negative test result who have CAD

198. Chronic reduction in coronary blood flow leading to decrease in contractile function that can be reversed by improving coronary flow is called:
   A. Hibernation
   B. Ischemia
   C. Infarction
   D. Stunning

199. Left ventricle (LV) ejection fraction (EF) reserve is defined as:
   A. Stress minus rest LVEF
   B. Stress minus rest LVEF/2
   C. Stress plus rest LVEF
   D. Stress plus rest LVEF/2

200. Which of the following results of the Duke Treadmill Scores (DTS) identifies patients with low risk CAD?
   A. ≤ -15
   B. -11 to -15
   C. $+4$ to -10
   D. $\geq +5$

201. A coronary angiogram of the right coronary artery (RCA) (Fig. 3.9) shows:
   A. 99 % lesion in the proximal RCA
   B. 50 % lesion in the proximal RCA
   C. 99 % lesion in the distal RCA
   D. 50 % lesion in the distal RCA

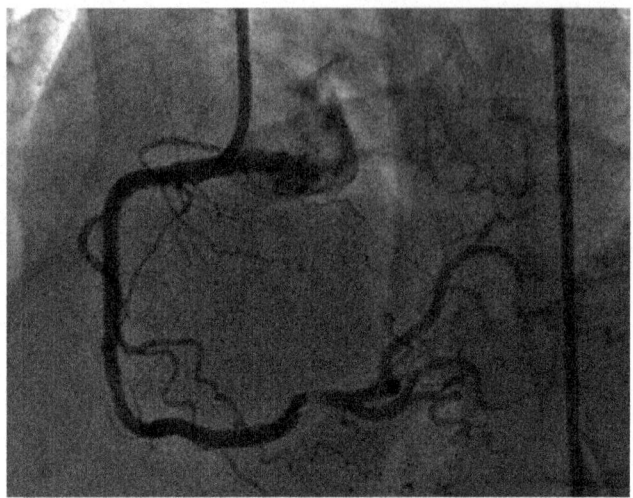

Fig. 3.9 Coronary angiogram

202. When semiquantitative approach is used to quantify MPI tracer uptake, the perfusion of each segment is scored according to a:
    A. 3-point scoring system
    B. 4-point scoring system
    C. 5-point scoring system
    D. 6-point scoring system

203. The rate of transfer of energy (LET) from ionizing radiation applied in diagnostic imaging is approximately:
    A. 1 keV per micron
    B. 3 keV per micron
    C. 6 keV per micron
    D. 9 keV per micron

204. The heart is enclosed in a double-walled sac called the:
    A. Endocardium
    B. Epicardium
    C. Myocardium
    D. Pericardium

205. Which of the following parameters describe the total of infarcted, ischemic, or jeopardized myocardium?
    A. Ejection Fraction (EF)
    B. Summed Stress Score (SSS)
    C. Summed Rest Score (SRS)
    D. Summed Difference Score (SDS)

206. A simple tool that facilitates the interpretation process of MPI by looking at all segments at once is called:
    A. Data base
    B. Polar map
    C. Snap shot
    D. Volume curve

207. Which of the following luminal diameter narrowing is considered likely to be hemodynamically significant?
    A. At least 3 % or greater
    B. At least 40 % or greater
    C. At least 50 % or greater
    D. At least 60 % or greater

208. 4D-MSPECT differs from QGS and ECTb software in defining the valve plane in the sense that it permits the mitral valve plane to move as much as:
    A. 6 mm inward toward the apex during systole
    B. 20 mm inward toward the apex during systole
    C. 6 mm outward toward the base during systole
    D. 20 mm outward toward the base during systole

209. Which of the following drugs is the most well-known cause of chemotherapy-induced cardiotoxicity?
    A. Actinomycin
    B. Adenosine
    C. Adriamycin
    D. Ampicillin

210. A 73-year-old male patient with a history of HTN and atypical chest pain. Describe cardiac CT findings:
    A. Normal LAD
    B. Stenotic LAD
    C. Normal LCX
    D. Stenotic LCX

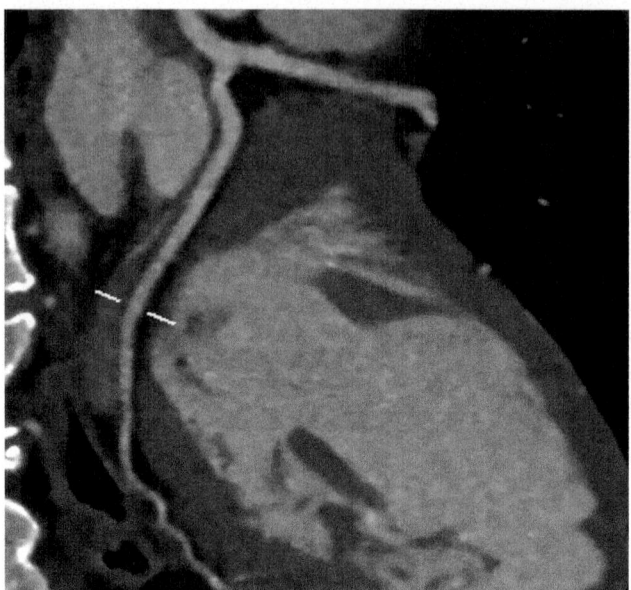

Fig. 3.10 Cardiac CT

211. Which of the following is the most common malignant primary cardiac tumor?
    A. Angiosarcoma
    B. Lipoma
    C. Melanoma
    D. Myxoma

212. The most common cause of syncope in the middle-aged are:
    A. Atrial arrhythmias
    B. Cardiac medications
    C. Neurocardiogenic disorders
    D. Ventricular arrhythmias

213. Tl-201 distributes proportionally to cardiac output in all tissues EXCEPT:
    A. Brain
    B. Liver
    C. Lung
    D. Muscles

214. For the first-pass acquisition, the gamma camera is placed in the shallow RAO position to maximize the likely separation of the:
    A. Left atrium and LV outflow tract
    B. Left atrium and RV outflow tract
    C. Right atrium and LV outflow tract
    D. Right atrium and RV outflow tract

215. All of the following are advantages of tomographic gated blood pool imaging (GBP) over planar GBP EXCEPT:
    A. Shorter processing time
    B. Higher contrast
    C. Simultaneous assessment of the right and left ventricles
    D. Three-dimensional localization

Answers

1. A. 5 min

   Peak myocardial concentration of thallium occurs within 5 min of injection. Following intravenous injection, about 5 % of the dose distributes to the myocardium, which extracts 80 to 90 % of the thallium as it passes through the coronary circulation.
   (Baggish and Boucher 2008)

2. B. Gadolinium-153

   As the scanning line source system moves and generates transmission images opposite the external source, images are simultaneously acquired through an electronic window in the detector that moves in a direction opposite to the line source.
   (Zaidi and Hasegawa 2003)

3. C. A dual-isotope technique

   Redistribution images from thallium can be obtained either at 4 h before the stress study or at 24 h after the 99mTc-99m activity has decayed. There is minimal redistribution of Tc-99m-based tracers compared with thallium.
   (Baggish and Boucher 2008)

4. C. Insulin stimulates cardiac F-18 FDG uptake; free fatty acids inhibit F-18 FDG accumulation

   Cardiac F-18 FDG uptake is strongly affected by metabolic conditions, in particular, by plasma levels of insulin and free fatty acids. Oral glucose loading and hyperinsulinemic euglycemic clamping can simulate these circumstances.
   (Schinkel et al. 2007)

5. D. Decreased levels of homocysteine

   Atherosclerotic plaque development results from multifaceted cellular interactions in the intima of arteries. This process takes place between resident cells of the vessel wall and cells of the immune system (leukocytes).
   (Strauss et al. 2004)

6. A. 1 %

   Patients with normal SPECT images had a lower risk of death and rate of hard cardiac events, while in patients with abnormal myocardial perfusion, the mortality and hard cardiac event rates are considerably higher. The only exceptions would appear to be patients with normal MPI in the presence of either a high risk treadmill ECG score or severe resting left ventricular dysfunction.
   (Gibbons 2000)

7. C. Dobutamine

Pharmacological stress agents fall into two categories: coronary vasodilating agents such as dipyridamole and adenosine and cardiac positive inotropic agents such as dobutamine—a sympathomimetic causing direct stimulation of $\beta1$ receptors of the sympathetic nervous system.
(Iskandrian et al. 2003)

8. A. Atrial fibrillation with rapid ventricular response

Atrial fibrillation occurs when many sites in the atria rapidly fire action potentials. The result is a Very fast atrial rate (f–f intervals can be shorter than 180 ms). The atrial action potentials all attempt to conduct through the AV node; however, the AV node becomes intermittently refractory and will only allow a certain number of atrial action potentials to reach the ventricles. This is why the ventricular rate is 3–4 times slower and completely irregular (no pattern) unless complete heart block or ventricular pacing is present.
(Goldberger 2006)

9. C. Transient ischemic dilation

The pathophysiology of a dilated, dysfunctional left ventricle during the stress is most likely related to sustained postischemic systolic dysfunction; evident dilation of the LV cavity represents diffuse subendocardial ischemia. There is relatively less tracer uptake in the subendocardium creating the appearance of an enlarged LV cavity.
(Zaret and Beller 2005)

10. C. Are higher in a supine position than in an upright position

With exercise, in healthy persons in supine positions, the elevation of cardiac output results almost exclusively from an increase in heart rate, with little increase of stroke volume.
(Bonow et al. 2011)

11. D. There is a temporal progression from hibernation to stunning

Research indicates that there is a temporal sequence from stunning, characterized by almost normal flow (with reduced flow reserve), to hibernation, with decreased resting flow.
(Schinkel et al. 2007)

12. D. 20–30° RAO

A shallow RAO view is recommended to improve right atrial–RV separation.
(ASNC Accessed Oct 22 2012)

13. A. lung uptake may be missed with Tc-99m tracers because of the more delayed onset of imaging compared with thallium

    Minimal background activity after thallium stress injection and the redistribution properties of Tl-201 dictate that imaging begin relatively early after stress, and as a result, lung uptake may be more apparent.
    (Bonow et al. 2011)

14. D. Time of flight

    Time of flight (TOF) takes advantage of very fast detectors and electronics that can measure the very short time difference (on the order of sub-nanoseconds) between the detection of each annihilation photon along the line of response between opposite detectors.
    (Bengel et al. 2009)

15. B. Apoptosis

    The cardiovascular pathologies of cardiomyopathy, heart failure, myocarditis, and myocardial infarction are associated with amplified levels of apoptosis, particularly in the myocyte.
    (Morrison and Sinusas 2009)

16. C. Technical factors—the camera is physically farther away from the septal myocardial wall

    During a SPECT acquisition, the camera is closer to the lateral myocardial wall than to the septum, resulting in less soft tissue attenuation and more efficient counts capture.
    (Bonow et al. 2011)

17. C. Dobutamine

    Dobutamine—the major inotropic/chronotropic agent—increases myocardial contractility, heart rate, and cardiac output, causing increased oxygen demand and consequential coronary vasodilation.
    (Zaret and Beller 2005)

18. A. Coronary flow reserve (CFR)

    CFR is the ratio of peak MBF during near maximal pharmacologically induced vasodilatation to resting MBF.
    (Schelbert 2009)

19. A. right coronary artery territory

    The RCA travels in the right atrio-ventricular (AIV) groove between the right atrium and right ventricle, as it wraps around to the inferior portion of the heart.
    (Zaret and Beller 2005)

20. B. 5 %

In general, oximetry is useful in monitoring *trending* of arterial oxygen satura-tion; a considerable desaturation should be confirmed with arterial blood gases.
(Bonow et al. 2011)

21. C. A doughnut artifact

The effects are most evident when the error is greater than two pixels in a 64 × 64 matrix. Errors less than this reduce spatial resolution, decrease image contrast through blurring of the image, and introduce significant artifacts (par-ticularly at the apex).
(Christian et al. 2004)

22. B. Early infarction

Depending on the residual degree of perfusion to the infarct zone, the test may not be positive for the first 24 h.
(Morrison and Sinusas 2009)

23. D. Decreased specificity

Attenuation artifact causes an increase in false-positive studies resulting in decreased specificity for the diagnosis of CHD and a decrease in the confi-dence of the referring and interpreting clinicians.
(Wheat and Currie 2004)

24. C. Oxygen-15-labeled (O-15) water

O-15-labeled water linearly tracks changes of myocardial blood flow.
(Schelbert 2009)

25. D. Hibernating myocardium

Chronic hibernation results from repeated episodes of reversible ischemia caused by a loss of coronary flow reserve that ultimately lead to a state of persistent postischemic dysfunction. Restoration of regional function after revascularization presupposes that revascularization successfully restores resting nutrient blood flow to normal levels, but inadequate revascularization can also be due to technical reasons.
(Gibbons 2000)

26. B. A reversible perfusion defect mimicking ischemia

Soft tissue attenuation artifacts caused by fixed anatomic structures are usu-ally present on both stress and rest images, if the position of the patient is the same during both acquisitions.
(Zaret and Beller 2005)

27. A. Restrict radiation dose

    The aim of justification, optimization, and limitation is to constrain the radia-
    tion dose so that doses to staff, patients, and the public stay below the level at
    which deterministic effects occur, and the probability of stochastic effects
    happening is limited to an acceptably low level.
    (ICRP 1991)

28. A. Decreases in proportion to the degree of stenosis severity

    In patients with CAD, CFR decreases in proportion to the degree of the sever-
    ity of the stenosis diameter.
    (Ghosh et al. 2010)

29. A. Attenuation artifacts from true perfusion defects

    Functional imaging may help in distinguishing between a prior myocardial
    infarction and attenuation artifact. Normal LV function in a region with a fixed
    defect on perfusion imaging can be categorized as a soft tissue attenuation
    artifact, whereas, abnormal function in conjunction with a similar fixed defect
    would indicate myocardial infarction or myocardial stunning.
    (Zaret and Beller 2005)

30. C. Premature atrial contractions

    Other unfavorable markers include ischemic changes in five or more electro-
    cardiographic leads and continuance of the changes in the late recovery phase
    of exercise.
    (Bonow et al. 2011)

31. B. Increased sensitivity and decreased resolution

    The thicker the crystal, the bigger the distribution of the emitted light photons
    produced from the scintillation, and the less precise the computation of gamma
    ray interaction location, thus causing poorer intrinsic resolution of the
    camera.
    (Christian et al. 2004)

32. D. Nitroglycerine

    Nitroglycerin is known to increase the blood supply to the myocardium and
    would thus increase the delivery of tracers to the tissue. The tracer concentration
    is an energy-dependent mechanism available only if the cells are still viable.
    (Ficaro and Hansen. Accessed Dec 13 2010)

33. C. Functional information

    ECG-gated imaging, also called functional imaging, may help differentiate
    between a myocardial infarction and an attenuation artifact.
    (Zaret and Beller 2005)

34. C. Oxygen-15–labeled (O-15) water

O-15-labeled water not only exchanges from the blood into the myocardium, but similarly equilibrates with the water spaces in blood, demanding corrections for tracer activity in the left ventricular blood pool and the vascular space of the myocardium.
(Schelbert 2009)

35. C. Cardiac catheterization

Cardiac catheterization is routinely used to correlate the findings of MPI; on the basis of catheterization, the patient is categorized as having CAD or not having CAD.
(Koller 2002)

36. C. Hyperventilation

As exercise becomes more intense, the surge in lactic acid becomes greater leading to metabolic acidosis. Formed lactate is buffered in the serum by the bicarbonate system, resulting in increased carbon dioxide excretion.
(Bonow et al. 2011)

37. A. Indirectly by inhibiting reuptake of adenosine

The biologic half-life of natural adenosine, normally 15–30 s in the bloodstream, increases with dipyridamole infusion, tripling or quadrupling the level of circulating adenosine.
(Iskandrian et al.2003)

38. B. Low rates of uptake of glucose and lactate and the high rates of uptake and oxidation of free fatty acid

The fed state is differentiated by high rates of uptake and oxidation of glucose and lactate and low FFA uptake.
(Ghosh et al. 2010)

39. C. Vertical long-axis view

The vertical long axis is displayed with serial slices beginning at the septum and progressing to the lateral wall of the left ventricle, the heart in a horizontal position and the cardiac apex to the viewer's right.
(SNM 1992)

40. D. Repolarization abnormalities

Over-reading of the computerized interpretation by the physician and comparison with previous tracings are mandatory.
(Goldman and Schafer 2012)

41. A. Decreased sensitivity

    Because of this resolution vs. sensitivity trade-off, the collimator is possibly the most significant piece of the SPECT camera affecting image characteristic.
    (Early and Sodee 1995)

42. B. Histogram

    Review of the beat-length R–R interval histogram can be used to assess cardiac rhythm abnormalities or determine if significant arrhythmias were present.
    (ASNC Accessed July 24, 2013)

43. C. Vertical long-axis view

    This orientation is similar to the orientation of a right anterior oblique to left ventriculogram.
    (SNM July 1992)

44. A. Rb-82 displays a nonlinear relationship between blood flow and myocardial activity concentrations

    Rb-82 displays tracer kinetic properties that are comparable to those of N-13 ammonia; however, its first-pass extraction fraction is lower than that of N-13 ammonia and as a result reaches the "plateau phase" at somewhat lower flows (i.e., 2.0–2.5 mL/min/g), when compared with N-13 ammonia (2.5–3.0 mL/min/g)
    (Schelbert 2009)

45. B. The aorta and the right atrium

    Coronary blood flow is dependent upon arterial pressure, diastolic time, and small vessel resistance. The system is regulated to achieve a low flow high oxygen extraction and low myocardial Po2. This setting is sensitive to change in oxygen needs.
    (Schelbert 2009)

46. B. Cut-off

    The cut-off value is defined as the frequency at which the filter value falls to 0.0; since some filters never have values of 0.0 for the frequencies we are interested in, the more convenient description of the cut-off is used.
    (Zubal and Wisniewski 1997)

47. C. Dobutamine

    Vasodilating agents operate directly on the coronary vessels to increase blood flow, while inotropic agents, e.g., dobutamine, work indirectly by increasing myocardial work load—for both, in the presence of coronary artery disease (CAD), perfusion image abnormalities result from heterogeneity of coronary blood flow reserve.
    (Iskandrian et al. 2003)

48. A. Shorten as heart rate increases

When the heart rate goes up, P amplitude increases, and the PR segment becomes increasingly more downsloping in the inferior leads.
(Hill and Timmis Accessed Nov 22 2012)

49. B. An active filter

Adaptive filters, named also as restorative or active filters, utilize some criteria from the resolution capabilities of the camera and collimator, and assimilate them into the mathematical filter function.
(Christian et al. 2004)

50. C. Fatigue

The most common motive for discontinuing an exercise test is fatigue and breathlessness
as a result of the unfamiliar exercise.
(Banerjee et al. 2012)

51. C. Gynecomastia

Gynecomastia is a benign enlargement of the male breast resulting from a proliferation of the glandular component of the breast.
(Frohlich 2001)

52. B. 25 ms

Ideally, the frame time should be adjusted to match the heart rate at the time of acquisition. To avoid the probable errors that might occur if the frame time was frequently being manipulated, a standard of 25 ms per frame is suggested for all acquisitions.
(ASNC Accessed June 17 2012)

53. D. A low pass filter

The flexibility and ease of scheme of Butterworth filters have made them the filters of choice in most nuclear medicine procedures.
(Christian et al. 2004)

54. C. Rest transmission scan, rest images, stress images, stress transmission scan

Positron images are generally corrected for attenuation. Because of the short physical half-life of Rb-82, and to minimize misalignment between emission and transmission images, pharmacologic stress is used.
(Takalkar et al. 2008)

55. D. Ventricular pacemaker

Ventricular pacing appears on the electrocardiogram as a single pacemaker spike, followed by a QRS complex that is wide, bizarre, and resembles a ventricular beat.
(Goldberger 2006)

56. C. Walking at 3–4 mph

Workloads of 5–7 METs are matched with exterior carpentry, playing singles tennis, and light backpacking; running at 6–7 mph is equivalent of more than 9 METs.
(Bonow et al. 2011)

57. D. Atropine

Atropine may help to reach the maximum heart rate on a dobutamine stress test, as dobutamine has a less than optimal chronotropic—change the heart rate—effect.
(Iskandrian et al. 2003)

58. B. The PQ junction

The TP segment corresponds to a true isoelectric point but is not a practical choice for most customary clinical measurements.
(Goldberger 2006)

59. B. The lateral myocardial wall

Small breasts that lie over the anterior chest wall may attenuate the anterior or anteroseptal walls of the myocardium.
(Manglos et al. 1993)

60. D. Septum

False-positive perfusion defects occur frequently during exercise myocardial perfusion studies in patients with left bundle branch block (LBBB), due to asynchronous ventricular contraction which worsens with exercise. Pharmacologic stress imaging with adenosine and dobutamine is associated with fewer false-positive septal perfusion defects (improved specificity) than exercise testing in patients with LBBB.
(Zaret and Beller 2005)

61. B. Tc-99m teboroxime

Tc-99m teboroxime is a neutral lipophilic boronic acid conjugated to technetium dioxime for cardiac imaging. The main disadvantage is rapid myocardial clearance that necessitates imaging immediately after injection and limits its versatility.
(Gibbons 2000)

62. B. Transient atrioventricular block

The isotope injection may result in a small bolus of adenosine being administered through the line, and transient, short-lived, and self-limited atrioventricular block can be observed.
(Miyamoto et al. 2007)

63. B. More rapid liver clearance

Tetrofosmin is similar to sestamibi in uptake and clearance properties. A more
rapid liver clearance of tetrofosmin often causes a greater cardiac-to-hepatic
ratio during standard cardiac imaging.
(Coakley et al. 1989)

64. D. Energy of 1.19 MeV and an average range of 0.4 mm

The physical characteristics of the positrons emitted by N-13 ammonia are
similar to that of F-18, and subsequently it produces excellent PET images.
Nitrogen N-13 decays to Carbon C 13 (stable) by positron emission and has a
physical half-life of 9.96 min. The principal photons useful for imaging are
the dual 511 keV gamma photons that are produced and emitted simultaneously in opposite direction when the positron interacts with an electron.
(Takalkar et al. 2011)

65. B. Nitric oxide

Nitric oxide (NO) is produced by many cells in the body; however, its production by vascular endothelium is particularly important in the regulation of
blood flow.
(Schelbert 2009)

66. A. 19 %

ESV(end systolic volume) is the amount of blood in the ventricle at the end of
the cardiac ejection period, and immediately preceding ventricular relaxation;
used as a measure of systolic function—usually about 50–60 mL, but sometimes as little as 10–30 mL in the normal.
(Zaret and Beller 2005)

67. D. Triggering of the A_{2A} adenosine receptor

Regadenoson is a low affinity agonist for the A_{2A} adenosine receptor, with at
least 10-fold lower
affinity for the A_1 adenosine receptor, and weak, if any, affinity for the A_{2B} and
A_3 adenosine receptors. The A_{2B} and A_3 adenosine receptors have been implicated in the pathophysiology of bronchoconstriction in predisposed individuals.
(Astellas Accessed July 28 2012)

68. C. 8 ml O_2/min per 100 g

    MVO_2 during heavy exercise can reach 70 ml O_2/min per 100 g; by comparison, the oxygen consumption for the kidney is 5 ml O_2/min per 100 g and for the brain is 3 ml O_2/min per 100 g.
    (Klabunde Accessed July 21 2012)

69. B. Increased BF in the normal territory and relatively unchanged BF in the territory supplied by the stenotic vessel

    Perfusion tracer administration in this setting demonstrates a defect in the area supplied by the stenotic vessel.
    (Dilsizian et al. 2009)

70. C. Metabolic equivalent (MET)

    Assessment of an individual's functioning against normal standards provides an estimate of the degree of exercise impairment.
    (Bonow et al. 2011)

71. A. The maximum myocardial tracer content

    This approach permits comprehensive and correct quantitative assessment of segmental tracer activity whenever the maximum myocardial tracer content (brightest pixel count) is located in the same myocardial region on the resting and the stress images.
    (Zaret and Beller 2005)

72. D. 45° LAO

    The LAO view is adjusted to visualize the septum, but the angle will be influenced by body habitus and cardiac orientation.
    (Zaret and Beller 2005)

73. D. Represents heterogeneity of flow between the LAD and left circumflex territories

    Since a septal defect in the left bundle branch block is most frequently observed at high heart rates, vasodilator stress is recommended in patients with LBBB.
    (Ficaro and Hansen Accessed May 22 2012)

74. B. Within a timing window and along a line of response

    Each annihilation produces two 511 keV photons travelling in opposite directions—180°±0.25° line of response (LOR)—and these photons may be detected if occurring within a certain time window —a timing window ~10 ns—and thus be determined to have come from the same annihilation.
    (Lin and Alavi 2009)

75. C. MPI findings

   Coronary artery disease (CAD) is the end result of the accumulation of atheromatous plaques within the walls of the coronary arteries that supply the
   myocardium
   (Fox et al. 2004)

76. D. Single-isotope MPI routinely assesses myocardial viability

   Although some studies have validated both Tc-99m sestamibi and tetrofosmin
   as equivalent to rest redistribution Tl-201 for the assessment of myocardial
   viability, single isotope studies are not routinely used for the assessment of
   myocardial viability.
   (Papaioannou and Heller Accessed July 22 2011)

77. C. B

   The LV counts are proportional to its volume, and the change from end-
   systolic counts to end-diastolic counts of the LV is used for the calculation of
   left ventricular ejection fraction.
   End-systolic volumes (ESV) or end-diastolic volumes (EDV) are more significant predictors of prognosis than EF, which is simply an arithmetical value
   based on these two parameters.
   (Zaret and Beller 2005)

78. B. 125 ms per frame

   1,000 ms/8 frame = B. 125 ms per frame
   (Zaret and Beller 2005)

79. D. Right ventricle overload

   The major changes in ventricular function as a result of pulmonary hypertension include right ventricular hypertrophy and dilatation, progressive volume
   overload, as well as right ventricular systolic dysfunction.
   (Zaret and Beller 2005)

80. C. Premature atrial contraction

   These changes should be recorded at least in three consecutive beats.
   (Iskandrian and Garcia 2012)

81. C. Dose extravasation

   A defect on the resting images can also appear more severe if the image scale
   factor has been changed due to tracer washout or higher visceral activity on
   resting acquisition.
   (Zaret and Beller 2005)

82. B. A microemboli in the brain

Although the possibility of producing microembolic cerebral infarctions is remote, it has been recommended to lower the number of particles injected to 10,000.
(Treves et al. 2007)

83. A. The hepatobiliary system

As a result, when performing cardiac imaging, there is often radioactivity present in the liver, gall bladder, and gastrointestinal tract from stomach to large bowel necessitating delay imaging. Sestamibi is taken up predominantly by passive cellular diffusion.
(Chamarthy and Travin 2010)

84. C. During the PET study

Motion during a scan results in blurred edges and loss of anatomic detail.
(Zaret and Beller 2005)

85. B. An overestimation of test sensitivity and an underestimation of test specificity

Nuclear cardiology referral bias, in which the result of a diagnostic test affects the subsequent referral for a more definitive test, influences the accuracy of noninvasive tests for coronary artery disease.
(Sica 2006)

86. B. Positron emission tomography

The reported PET scanning sensitivity and specificity are ~91 and 82% accordingly.
(Papaioannou and Heller Accessed July 22 2011)

87. B. 1–4 min after injection of Lexiscan

The half-life of this initial phase is approximately 2–4 min.
(Astellas Accessed July 28 2012)

88. C. Diastolic filling

The assessment of left ventricular (LV) diastolic function should be an integral part of a routine examination, particu-larly in patients presenting with dyspnea or heart failure.
(Zaret and Beller 2005)

89. A. Solid-state detectors

High resolution Cadmium Zinc Telluride (CZT) semiconductor radiation detectors—first flown on the successful NASA SWIFT mission in 2004; they are enabling a new generation of high performance detection and imaging equipment including Nuclear Cardiology.
(Christian et al. 2004)

90. B. Achieved 85 % of the maximum predicted heart rate, D. No ST segment depression

E. A physiological response in blood pressure
In most laboratories, test interpretation is based primarily on ST-segment changes, exercise-induced angina, and exercise capacity.
(Banerjee et al. 2012)

91. C. 30 % and 15 %

The lower energy and greater width of the Tl-201 photopeak requires a wider energy window.
(Holly et al. 2010)

92. B. Electronically paced rhythms

C. Left bundle branch block
Patients who have exercise limitations, and who have contraindications to vasodilator stress testing, can be referred for a pharmacologic stress test with dobutamine.
(ASNC. Accessed April 07 2012)

93. D. A negative test result who have CAD

True negative (TN) refers to patients with a negative test result who do not have CAD.
(Koller 2002)

94. 94. D. Dobutamine

Dobutamine augments myocardial contractility, heart rate, and cardiac output, resulting in increased oxygen demand and secondary coronary vasodilation.
(Zaret and Beller 2005)

95. C. 70 % or greater diameter reduction

The extent of disease is usually defined as 1-vessel, 2-vessel, 3-vessel, or left main disease.
(Scanlon et al. 1999)

96. D. Septal wall (Fig. 3.11)

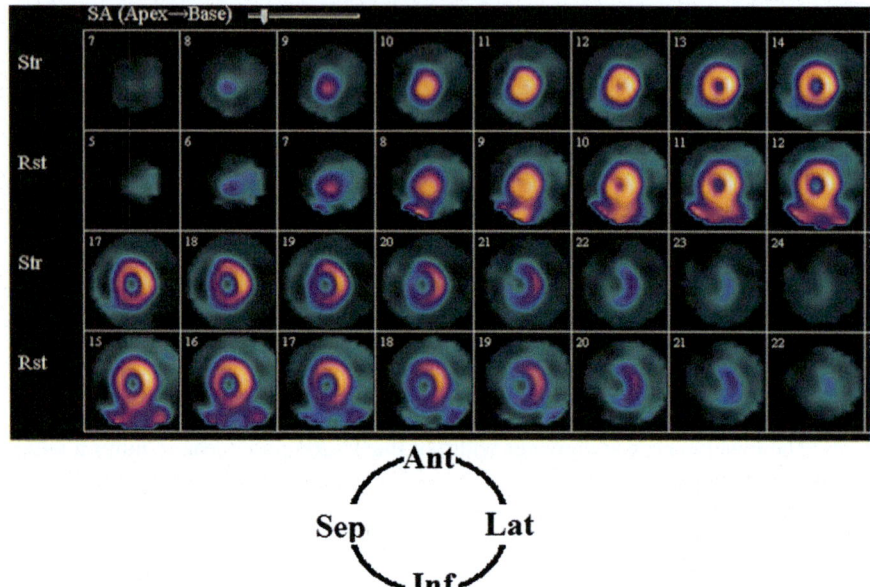

Fig. 3.11 SPECT MPI

97. B. 8–10 mSV

Radiation exposure is an essential consideration in the determination of which stress protocol to use in the laboratory, and for this reason the use of technetium for either stress-only imaging or rest/stress imaging is advocated. (Cerqueira et al. 2010)

98. C. 120 ml

End-diastolic volume (EDV) is the volume of blood in the right and/or left ventricle at end load or filling in (diastole). Normal range: 65–240 ml. (Schlosser et al. 2005)

99. D. patients in the selected high-intermediate or high risk population

A selective stress-only imaging strategy has potential to improve patient flow and laboratory utilization, and save time, radiation dose, and cost. (Des Prez et al. 2009)

100. A. Aggrenox

Atrial repolarization—may extend into the ST segment and T wave—and resting ST depression also decrease the diagnostic accuracy of the exercise ECG. (Akinpelu Accessed Oct 11 2012)

101. B. Hg-201

Thallium has 25 isotopes; Tl-204 is the most stable radioisotope, with a half-life of 3.78 years.
(Early and Sodee 1995)

102. A. regadenoson has a longer half-life than adenosine

Regadenoson, an adenosine analog, produces hyperemia with rapid onset (30 s) for a longer period (approximately, 2–5 min) than adenosine, which permits more convenient administration (injection over 10 s)
(Akinpelu Accessed Oct 11 2012)

103. D. Patients with high pretest probability of disease

The clinician's knowledge and experience, and the clinical presentation, are used to determine the patient's pretest likelihood of CAD. This pretest measure is evaluated on the basis of patient history, physical examination, and risk factor assessment.
(Weiner Accessed July 02 2012)

104. B. 2D PET

The 2D arrangement not only minimizes out-of-plane randoms or scatter events but also eliminates many true counts, thus reducing sensitivity.
(Lin and Alavi 2009)

105. B. Oxygen consumption of the heart

Oxygen consumption by the heart can be estimated by using the Fick Principle, which requires catheterization of the coronary sinus to measure venous oxygen saturation and coronary blood flow. Relative changes in MVO_2 can be estimated by using an indirect index such as the pressure-rate product.
(Klabunde Accessed July 21 2012)

106. B. Reverse redistribution

Currently, the pathophysiology and clinical significance of reverse redistribution phenomenon remain controversial. Reverse redistribution on SPECT does not appear to be an unfavorable prognostic factor in patients with chest pain.
(Zaret and Beller 2005)

107. B. An increase in heart rate and a decrease in blood pressure

Hemodynamic effects observed within 45 min of regadenoson administration—increase in heart rate and a decrease in blood pressure—are similar to adenosine.
(Astellas Accessed July 28 2012)

108. B. Patients with evidence of CAC and abnormal SPECT MPI

Information from the two testing modalities is complementary in the sense of the ability to refine risk predictions about outcomes and potentially tailoring the aggressiveness of secondary prevention. Studies are ongoing in this regard. (Berman et al. 2006)

109. B. Within 6 h of preparation

The combination of sestamibi and Tc-99m is shaken exuberantly, boiled for 10 min, and then cooled at room temperature for 15 min. It must then be used within 6 h of preparation.
(Baggish and Boucher 2008)

110. A. Exercise echocardiography

Echocardiography is mainly indicated in patients with abnormal resting ECGs (LBBB, LVH, digoxin effect, etc.), when the ECG is not sufficient to identify ischemia.
(Armstrong and Ryan 2008)

111. B. 89 % and 75 %, respectively

Sensitivities (generally uncorrected for referral bias) average 87 % and 89 %, respectively; specificities (also uncorrected) average 73 % and 75 %.
(ACC/AHA/ASNC Accessed July 24 2012)

112. A. Tc-99m MAA

Tc-99m albumin aggregate particles are efficiently trapped by the pulmonary capillaries such that usually only about 3 % of the activity is seen outside the lungs. When there is a right-to-left shun, some of the MAA escapes from the pulmonary circulation and lodges in the systemic capillaries.
(MacDonald and Burrell 2008)

113. C. Attenuation

Patient tissue between the radioactive material and the detector can substantially reduce the radiation reaching the detector, e.g., for Tc-99m, a soft tissue thickness of approximately 4.5 cm will reduce the intensity to one-half.
(Parker et al. 1984)

114. B. 140 µg/kg per min for 6 min

Adenosine should be given as a continuous peripheral intravenous infusion— half-life of adenosine is less than 10 s. Concurrent low level treadmill exercise during adenosine infusion is safe, well tolerated and results in fewer side effects, and improves image quality.
(Heller et al. Accessed July 22 2011)

115. B. Diastolic blood pressure greater than 90 mmHg

Cholesterol greater than 240 mg/dL, systolic blood pressure greater than 140 mmHg, smoking, diabetes, and family history of heart attack or sudden cardiac death in a first-degree relative younger than 60 years are multiple risk factors for CAD.
(Akinpelu Accessed Oct 11 2012)

116. A. Patients with coronary artery disease

When a patient is incapable to conclude moderate levels of exercise, or reach at least 85 %–90 % of age-predicted maximum, the level of exercise achieved may be inadequate to test cardiac reserve.
(Froelicher and Myers 2006)

117. C. sinus rhythm with frequent PVC in a pattern of bigeminy

Bigeminy describes a heart arrhythmia in which abnormal heart beats follow every other concurrent beat. In the absence of heart disease, premature ventricular complexes are associated with little or no increased risk of developing a dangerous arrhythmia. The episode of PVCs in patients with structural heart disease has been shown to considerably increase the risk of subsequent morbidity and mortality
(Goldberger 2006)

118. C. A high coronary calcium score implies severe stress-induced perfusion abnormalities

The presence of even extensive CAC does not always represent obstructive stenosis resulting in stress-induced perfusion abnormalities; stress SPECT MPI is an appropriate test to perform to evaluate the need for and potential benefit of catheterization and revascularization.
(Brindis et al. 2005)

119. D. Motion of 2 pixels

Motion of 0.5 pixel is usually not visually detectable; 1 pixel of motion was recognized but judged to be clinically insignificant; 2 pixels of motion led to clinically significant artifacts in 5 % of interpretations.
(Cooper et al. 1992)

120. B. A non-diagnostic test

Failure to reach that heart rate target leads to a test being labeled as "nondiagnostic" or "submaximal" but not necessarily abnormal.
(Lauer 2001)

121. C. An attenuation map

The attenuation maps are integrated with the raw myocardial perfusion images to reconstruct image data with attenuation correction.
(Zaidi and Hasegawa 2003)

122. D. Systolic blood pressure more than 90 mmHg

Patients with an SBP less than 90 mmHg should not undertake adenosine stress testing because of the potential for further lowering of the blood pressure.
(Akinpelu Accessed Oct 02 2012)

123. D. Patients with severe ischemia

In patients with severe ischemia, redistribution may be very slow and may take more than 4 h—reinjection at rest may improve sensitivity for the detection of viability.
(Zaret and Beller 2005)

124. B. Increased sensitivity

PET sensitivity is greater by approximately two to three orders of magnitude; single-photon imaging (planar and SPECT) use physical collimators to reject photons.
(Rahmima and Zaidib 2008)

125. C. The right atrium, the lung, the left atrium

Blood from the body leaves the systemic circulation when it enters the right atrium through the superior vena cava and the inferior vena cava and then is pumped through the tricuspid valve into the right ventricle. From the RV, blood travels through the lungs, leaves the lungs through the pulmonary veins, enters the left atrium, which pumps it through the mitral valve and then into the left ventricle, and from there the blood is pumped out into the aorta and the entire systemic circulation.
(Frohlich 2001)

126. D. Time of acquisition

The CDR is also influenced by septal scatter, which is caused by photons that scatter in the collimator septa and still remain within the detection energy window.
(Rahmima and Zaidib 2008)

127. C. Dyspnea, headache

Most adverse reactions began soon after dosing, and generally resolved within approximately 15 min, except for headaches which resolved in most patients within 30 min.
(Astellas Accessed July 28 2012)

128. C. Ischemic cardiomyopathy

The term ischemic cardiomyopathy has been used to describe significantly impaired left ventricular function (left ventricular ejection fraction ≤35–40 %) that results from coronary artery disease.
(Fang Accessed June 10 2012)

129. C. Directly proportional to the width and inversely proportional to the length of the collimator hole

Collimator resolution constitutes the major part of the overall spatial resolution and primarily arises from the collimator design.
(DePuey 2012)

130. B. +4 to −10

Approximately, 70 % of the patients in the intermediate Duke Treadmill Score category had a normal stress perfusion study, associated with a very low risk natural history.
(Mark et al. 1987)

131. C. Attenuation correction

In order for the CT image to be employed in the attenuation correction algorithm, the CT numbers (in Hounsfield units, HU) must be adapted to attenuation coefficients at the energy of the SPECT radionuclide.
(Kinahan et al. 1998)

132. D. Vertical

In the appropriate LAO view, the long axis is vertical, the apex is pointing down, and left ventricle is on the right side of the image.
(Zaret and Beller 2005)

133. C. Reduce image accuracy

Tl-201 is continually exchanged between the extracellular and intracellular spaces; this exchange is dependent on the degree of blood flow to the region of interest, which can result in resolution of stress-related perfusion differences in as little as 20 or 30 min if, for this reason, imaging should begin within 10–15 min after peak stress injection.
(Baggish and Boucher 2008)

134. D. Sodium iodide activated with thallium

The sodium iodide activated with thallium NaI(Tl) crystal was exploited in the original PET scanners, but its density was too low to have effective stopping power for 511 keV photons.
(Lin and Alavi 2009)

135. A. Dilated cardiomyopathy

A normal heart has a LVEF of ~50–65 %. In patients with dilated cardiomy-opathy (DCM), the contractility of the heart is severely impaired, leading to systolic dysfunction. Typical LVEFs in end-stage DCM are in the range of 25–40 %

(Kumar et al. 2009)

136. B. Resolution

For projection data acquired with an Anger camera, the total resolution depends on the intrinsic resolution and the collimator resolution.

(Early and Sodee 1995)

137. C. Perpendicular to the long axis of the left ventricle

The benefits of reorientation involve easier visual evaluation of myocardial perfusion defects and the capability to more precisely quantify and display perfusion parameters.

(Germano and Berman 2006)

138. A. High rates of uptake and oxidation of glucose and lactate and the low rates of uptake of free fatty acid

The fasting state is differentiated by low rates of uptake of glucose and lactate and the high rates of uptake and oxidation of free fatty acid.

(Ghosh et al. 2010)

139. B. The myocardial perfusion at the time of injection and the LV function at the time of acquisition

Since sestamibi or tetrofosmin exhibit minimal redistribution, in healthy sub-jects, poststress gated images represent stress perfusion and a resting state function. On the other hand, in patients with severe ischemia, stress-induced LV dysfunction may be continued for a prolonged period (a weakened func-tion during the poststress acquisition may be detected when compared with the resting measurement).

(Paul and Nabi 2004)

140. B. 2.5 mph

The treadmill is started at 2.74 km/h (1.7 mph) and at a gradient (or incline) of 10 %. The protocol has seven stages, each lasting 3 min, resulting in 21 min' exercise for a complete test.

(Hill Accessed June 09 2012)

141. B. 17-segment model

The 17-segment model delivers the most accurate agreement with the available anatomic data, and has the best fit; for this reason, 17-segment model is commonly used in both echocardiography and SPECT nuclear cardiology.
(Cerqueira et al. 2002)

142. A. A 2-dimensional snapshot of the 3-dimensional distribution of radioactivity

The result of tomographic image reconstruction is 2-dimensional images that are perpendicular to the long axis of the human body, with each of these images corresponding to a specific 2-dimensional slice of the body.
(Germano 2001)

143. C. Exercise ECG

Since the resting ECG is normal and interpretable, appropriate use criteria recommend exercise ECG over stress radionuclide myocardial perfusion imaging.
(Hendel et al. 2009)

144. B. Fatty acid metabolism

Fatty acid metabolism imaging has great potential in diagnosis and monitoring of patients with ischemic heart disease, cardiomyopathies, myocarditis, acute coronary syndrome, and heart failure.
(Ghosh et al. 2010)

145. C. Higher left than right ventricle pressure

Ventricular septal defect defines one or more holes in the wall that separates the right and left ventricles of the heart. It is one of the most common congenital heart defects.
(MacDonald and Burrell 2008)

146. C. True perfusion abnormalities

Concern regarding the production of artifacts on the other hand may correspondingly lead to an underinterpretation of true perfusion abnormalities, because the effects of soft tissue attenuation may be overemphasized by the reader.
(Burrell and MacDonald 2006)

147. C. A mild to moderate reduction in mean BP associated with a reflex increase in HR

Adenosine produces a direct negative chronotropic, dromotropic, and inotropic effect on the heart, and produces peripheral vasodilation—the net hemodynamic effect of adenosine in humans is in general a mild to moderate reduction in systolic, diastolic, and mean arterial blood pressure associated with a reflex increase in heart rate.
(Astellas Accessed March 28 2012)

148. D. Left bundle branch block

Reverse mismatch with LBBB has been suggested to be a consequence of altered septal glucose metabolism; this pattern can be observed also in patients with non-ischemic cardiomyopathy, repetitive stunning, following revascularization early post-MI, and in some patients with diabetes.
(Thompson et al. 2006)

149. D. Temporal blurring

Beat-rejection software allows to acquire data with a stable R–R interval based on the average of multiple R–R intervals before the acquisition and to specify a range of acceptable beats ("acceptance window").
(Paul and Nabi 2004)

150. D. Horizontal long-axis view

This orientation is similar to that of the transthoracic two-dimensional echocardiographic apical four-chamber view as displayed with the apex up.
(SNM 1992)

151. C. kiloelectronvolt per micron

Linear energy transfer (LET) is the average amount of energy a particular radiation imparts to the local medium per unit length.
(Statkiewicz-Sherer et al. 2011)

152. C. The potential for repeated assessment of cardiac function

Advantages of the equilibrium techniques are the potential for repeated assessment of cardiac function, high count density, and acquisition of images in multiple projections.
(Bonow et al. 2011)

153. B. Beats having duration of 0.72–0.88 s

The duration of one cardiac cycle in a subject with an average heart rate of 72 beats per minute is 0.8 s.
(Paul and Nabi 2004)

154. C. Depicts tracer kinetics

High temporal resolution allows for creation of dynamic imaging sequences to describe tracer kinetics.
(Bengel et al. 2009)

155. A. Angiogenesis

Angiogenesis seems to be stimulated by external processes, such as ischemia, hypoxia, inflammation, and shear stress.
(Fam et al. 2003)

156. B. Acute myocardial infarction (>2 days)

Acute myocardial infarction (<2 days), high-risk unstable angina, decompensated heart failure, uncontrolled cardiac arrhythmias with symptoms or hemodynamic compromise, advanced atrioventricular block, severe symptomatic aortic stenosis, and severe hypertrophic obstructive cardiomyopathy are also absolute contraindications to exercise testing.
(Bonow et al. 2011)

157. D. Cell membranes

The uptake and retention of these tracers do reflect regional flow differences, but myocyte cell membrane integrity is also a prerequisite.
(Dilsizian et al. 2009)

158. A. Atrioventricular node

The electrical relay station, atrioventricular (AV) node, between the upper and lower chambers of the heart decelerates the electrical current sent by the sinoatrial (SA) node before the signal is permitted to pass down through to the ventricles.
(Bonow et al. 2011)

159. D. Be excreted completely via urinary tract

The ideal perfusion tracer should follow myocardial blood flow across the complete physiologically significant range of blood flow; additionally, changes such as ischemia or medications should not interfere with its uptake so that the resulting regional tracer concentrations reflect myocardial perfusion.
(Dilsizian et al. 2009)

160. A. Nitroglycerine

Nitrates therapy decrease the size of reversible perfusion defects—nitroglycerin could limit or prevent the occurrence of ischemia during the exercise MPI. If MPI is performed for the primary diagnosis of CAD, or for reasons of initial risk stratification, anti-ischemic drugs should be withheld, though this should be done only if approved by the referring physician.
(Heller and Hendel 2011)

161. A. The higher dose is 3.5–4.0 times the lower dose

When a ratio 3:1 is employed, a 3- to 4-h delay between rest imaging and stress imaging allows radioactivity to decay by 29 %–37 %, thereby providing better image contrast.
(Van Train et al. 1994)

162. A. A1

Adenosine A2b receptors are present in bronchioles and the peripheral vasculature.
(Dilsizian et al. 2009)

163. B. Degradation of image contrast

With the stress–rest series, the rest activity may mask some of the stress defects, leading to the degradation of image contrast and a decrease in the detection of true reversibility.
(Husain 2007)

164. D. 4 mm, 10–12 mm

The spatial resolution of a PET scanner is a measure of the ability of the device to faithfully reproduce the image of an object, thus clearly depicting the variations in the distribution of radioactivity in the object.
(Pichler et al. 2008)

165. D. Stunning

The only correct way to diagnose stunning is to re-image the patient more than a few months after the original scan to visualize stunning reversibility.
(Zaret and Beller 2005)

166. C. Is the same among women and men

According to data from a meta-analysis, the mean sensitivity and specificity for SPECT MPI to detect coronary stenosis $\geq$50 % in women were 85 % and 79 % accordingly; for men, the sensitivity and specificity were similar at 89 % and 72 %, respectively.
(Iskandar et al. 2012)

167. A. Deterministic effect

Deterministic effects are described as having a threshold dose below which the effect is not distinguished. The seriousness of the effect increases with dose and dose rate.
(Lombardi 1999)

168. B. Patients with abnormal MPI are referred to coronary angiography

In its ultimate form, in which only patients with an abnormal test are referred for angiography, posttest referral bias drives the specificity to zero (there are no true-negatives).
(Ficaro and Hansen Accessed May 22 2012)

169. C. Endocardial contour

In patients with an uncompromising perfusion defect, large aneurysmal dilatation, or substantial structural distortion of the LV, the edge detection is often erroneous.
(Paul and Nabi 2004)

170. C. Hypovolemic, E. Physically deconditioned, F. In atrial fibrillation

The prognostic significance of an early abnormal increase of heart rate during low-level exercise is debatable.
(Chaitman 2007)

171. C. Tuning fork artifact

The accuracy of COR alignment should be checked weekly for each camera head, unless indicated otherwise by the manufacturer. If no specific COR acquisition protocol is recommended by the manufacturer, the COR can be determined through the acquisition of a point source of activity (18–37 MBq) on the patient table 4–8 in. away from the axis of rotation.
(Christian et al. 2004)

172. A.Tc-99m MAA

Tc-99m albumin aggregate particles are efficiently trapped by the pulmonary capillaries such that usually only about 3 % of the activity is seen outside the lungs. If there is a right-to-left shunt, some of the MAA outflows from the pulmonary circulation to the systemic capillaries. By comparing the counts in the lungs and in the systemic circulation, it is possible to assess the size of the right-to-left shunt.
(MacDonald and Burrell 2008)

173. D. Septal wall (Fig. 3.12)

(Zaret and Beller 2005)

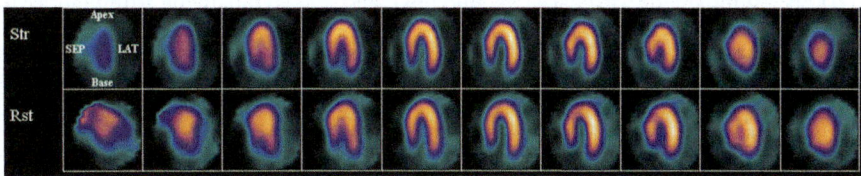

Fig. 3.12 SPECT MPI

174. C. Enhances renal excretion

Tc-99m DTPA and Tc-99m pertechnetate have short intravascular residence time; however, Tc-99m DTPA is the advised radionuclide of choice because the DTPA salt enhances renal excretion.
(Bonow et al. 2011)

175. A. Angiogenesis

Radiolabeled VEGF121 has been used to effectively identify angiogenesis in a rabbit model of hindlimb ischemia (produced by femoral artery ligation).
(Lu et al. 2003)

176. A. Chronotropic incompetence

Chronotropic incompetence or abnormal heart rate reserve results from decreased heart rate sensitivity to the normal increase in sympathetic tone during exercise.
(Froelicher and Myers 2006)

177. B. Necrosis

In-111 Antimyosin uptake is associated with the (WBC migration).
(Zaret and Beller 2005)

178. B. ~ 40 % of all deaths

Coronary artery disease, stroke, and congestive heart failure are responsible for 77 % of all cardiovascular deaths.
(Strauss et al. 2004)

179. C. A greater amount of tracer uptake in the septum relative to the lateral wall

The polar map display can create the impression of a mild lateral wall perfusion defect in patients diagnosed with HCM.
(Ficaro and Hansen 2012)

180. B. Sympathetic discharge is maximal and parasympathetic stimulation is withdrawn

Sympathetic discharge and withdraw of parasympathetic stimulation cause vasoconstriction of most circulatory body systems, except for that in exercising muscle, and in the cerebral and coronary circulations.
(Bonow et al. 2011)

181. C. Has no effect on diagnostic accuracy

The more favorable hyperemic stress accomplished with pharmacologic stress is counterbalanced by the lack of linear tracer uptake in the areas with the highest flow (the "roll-off" phenomenon of the common perfusion tracers).
(Dilsizian et al. 2009)

182. C. The coronary vasodilator effects would be reversed

Side effects from vasodilator pharmacologic stress, although common, in most circumstances may be tolerated; with more severe side effects, such as severe shortness of breath or bronchospasm, or with more dramatic ST-segment abnormalities, reversal of the dipyridamole effect more quickly might be required.
(Dilsizian et al. 2009)

183. B. Maximal coronary flow reserve is not achieved as often as with vasodilator pharmacologic stress

Dobutamine is suggested only when adenosine, dipyridamole, or regadenoson is contraindicated, e.g., in a patient with significant reactive airways disease. (Dilsizian et al. 2009)

184. B. Positron emitter germanium-68 or a single-photon emitter cesium-137

The rod rotates at a fixed speed in the gantry, and total coincident counts are measured without the patient (the blank scan), and repeated with the patient in the gantry (the transmission scan). (Bonow et al. 2011)

185. B. Cardiogenic shock

Cardiogenic shock is a major, and frequently fatal, complication of a variety of acute and chronic disorders, occurring most commonly following acute myocardial infarction (MI). (Lenneman et al. Accessed May 21 2012)

186. B. The amount of preserved tissue

The probability of functional recovery after revascularization is related to the magnitude of tracer uptake within that territory. (Bonow et al. 2011)

187. B. Contrast

Contrast is defined as the difference between the darkest and brightest peaks of the image. (Zubal and Wisniewski 1997)

188. C. Coronary artery disease

Distinguishing if LV dysfunction is the consequences of CAD is a critical early step in the management of patients with heart failure—a normal stress MPI scan is highly predictive for the absence of CAD. (Gheorghiade et al. 2006)

189. B. Patients with low pretest probability of disease

The American College of Cardiology has established guidelines for determining the pretest likelihood of CAD in patients with chest pain, according to their sex, age, and type of chest discomfort. Patients with a pretest likelihood of less than 15 % are considered to be at low risk for CAD, between 15 % and 85 % at moderate risk, and greater than 85 % at high risk. (Weiner Accessed July 02 2012)

190. B. The Duke treadmill score

This treadmill score has been shown to stratify prognosis accurately for both inpatient and outpatient ischemic heart disease populations.
(Mark et al. 1987)

191. C. Brighter and thicker

Tracer concentration within the myocardium is constant during a gated SPECT image acquisition. The recovery of counts (and thus the brightness of the object being imaged) is related to wall thickness.
(Bonow et al. 2011)

192. D. Valium

Labeling efficiency is also diminished when "old" Tc-99m-pertechnetate of low specific activity is used. Tc-99m decays to Tc-99, which is no longer useful for imaging, but contests with the radioactive form of stannous ions.
(ASNC Accessed June 17 2012)

193. C. Planar imaging has more ability to differentiate smaller perfusion abnormalities

As a result of the two-dimensional nature of planar imaging, there is significant overlap of myocardial regions resulting in less ability to differentiate smaller and milder perfusion defects.
(Germano and Berman 2006)

194. D. Projection line

As soon as each projection line has been corrected for attenuation, the emission data may be reconstructed into attenuation corrected emission image for clinical interpretation.
(Bonow et al. 2011)

195. B. 50 ml

End-systolic volume (ESV) is the volume of blood in a ventricle at the end of contraction, or systole, and the beginning of filling, or diastole. Normal range 16–143 ml
(Schlosser et al. 2005)

196. C. Gated projection data require more smoothing than ungated data

As a result of the relatively poor counts, gated projection data necessitate more smoothing than ungated or summed data during the reconstruction.
(Paul and Nabi 2004)

197. C. A positive test result who do not have CAD

   True positive (TP) refers to patients with a positive test result who have CAD.
   (Koller 2002)

198. A. Hibernation

   Ischemia, stunning, and hibernating refer to reversible tissue; myocardial
   infarction exemplifies irreversible tissue state.
   (Zaret and Beller 2005)

199. A. Stress minus rest LVEF

   LV ejection fraction reserve provides significant independent and incremental
   values for predicting future adverse events.
   (Dorbala et al. 2009)

200. D. $\geq +5$

   The typical observed range of DTS is from −25 (highest risk) to +15 (lowest risk).
   (Mark et al. 1987)

201. C. 99 % lesion in the distal RCA (Fig. 3.13)

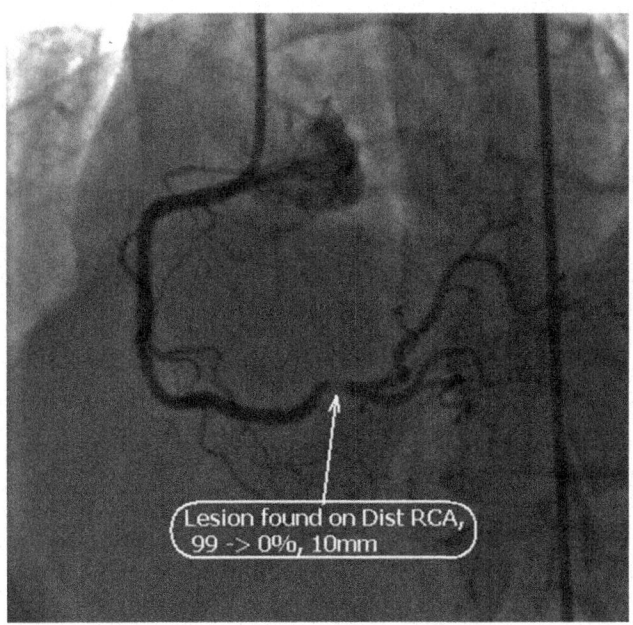

Fig. 3.13 Coronary angiogram

202. C. 5-point scoring system

     0—normal, 1—equivocal reduction, 2—definite but moderate reduction, 3—
     severe reduction of tracer uptake, 4—absent uptake of radioactivity
     (Khalil 2011)

203. B. 3 keV per micron

     X-rays and gamma rays are highly penetrating radiations and as such do not
     easily give up their energy and are considered low LET radiations.
     (Statkiewicz-Sherer et al. 2011)

204. D. Pericardium

     The heart is enclosed in a double-walled sac called the pericardium: the outer
     wall, called the pericardial sac (parietal pericardium), and visceral pericar-
     dium covering the heart surface.
     (Saladin 2009)

205. B. Summed Stress Score (SSS)

     Summed Stress Score (SSS) is the total segmental scores of stress images. The
     summed scores are to perfusion what the ejection fraction index is to ventricu-
     lar function.
     (Fuster et al. 2007)

206. B. Polar map

     Polar map also provides a measure of defect reversibility based on normaliz-
     ing the rest images with the stress images and color-coding scheme.
     (Khalil 2011)

207. C. At least 50 % or greater

     Resistance through a stenosis depends on many variables including length and
     morphology—so this is only a rough indication.
     (Ho and Reddy 2011)

208. B. 20 mm inward toward the apex during systole

     If serial EF assessments are being performed, the accuracy of the estimates is
     reduced by using the basal range of (0, 6) mm rather than (5,20) mm. Corridor
     4DM allows the user to set the range of motion—5 mm and 20 mm from end
     diastole (ED) to end systole—for the valve plane.
     (Ficaro et al. 2003)

209. C. Adriamycin

     The anthracyclines, daunorubicin (Cerubidine, Daunomycin), doxorubicin
     (Adriamycin, Rubex), and idarubicin (Idamycin) and epirubicin are the most
     likely cause of cardiovascular complications in oncology patients. Chronic
     cardiomyopathy is the most severe form of doxorubicin cardiotoxicity.
     (Pharmacotherapeutics Accessed Sept 23 2012)

210. C. Normal LCX

   The left main coronary artery (LM) originates from the left coronary sinus of Valsalva and gives origin to the left anterior descending coronary artery (LAD) and left circumflex coronary artery (LCX) in the atrioventricular (AV) groove. (Saladin 2009)

211. A. Angiosarcoma

   An angiosarcoma is an uncommon—autopsy prevalence of 0.001–0.28 %—malignant neoplasm characterized by rapidly proliferating, extensively infiltrating anaplastic cells derived from blood vessels. A myxoma is the most common of all benign heart tumors. (Bonow et al. 2011)

212. C. Neurocardiogenic

   Neurally mediated syncopal syndrome includes carotid sinus syndrome, situational syncope, and neurocardiogenic syncope (also known as vasovagal syncope). (Strickberger et al. 2006)

213. A. Brain

   Tl-201 distributes proportionately to cardiac output in all tissues except brain (as a result of intact blood–brain barrier) and fat. Blood–brain barrier is best portrayed as a physical and metabolic barrier with selective transport systems acting as a signaling interface between brain and blood. (Weissleder et al. 2011)

214. D. right atrium and RV outflow tract

   With this technique, right ventricular ejection fraction (RVEF) is derived from a right ventricular activity vs time curve. FP is much less commonly used in clinical practice because of the emergence of alternative techniques. (Ho and Reddy 2011)

215. A. shorter processing time

   GBP SPECT features analysis of RV and LxV contraction phase information, in contrast to gated MPI phase analysis, which presently measures only contraction phases for the left ventricle, but not for the right ventricle. (Chen et al. 2008)

References and Suggested Readings

ACC/AHA/ASNC Guidelines for the clinical use of cardiac radionuclide imaging—executive summary. http://circ.ahajournals.org/content/108/11/1404.full#sec-1.

Akinpelu D ed. Treadmill stress testing http://emedicine.medscape.com/article/1827089. Accessed Oct 11 2012

Armstrong WF, Ryan T. Stress echocardiography from 1979 to present. J Am Soc Echocardiogr. 2008;21:22.

ASNC.http://www.asnc.org/imageuploads/ImagingGuidelinesFPRNA020509.pdf.

ASNC. Pharmacologic and exercise stress tests. http://www.asnc.org/media/PDFs/PPStressTests081511.pdf.

Astellas. http://www.astellas.us/docs/lexiscan.pdf.

Baggish LA, Boucher AC. Radiopharmaceutical agents for myocardial perfusion imaging. Circulation. 2008;118:1668–74.

Banerjee A, Newman DR, Van den Bruel A, Heneghan C. Diagnostic accuracy of exercise stress testing for coronary artery disease: a systematic review and meta-analysis of prospective studies. Int J Clin Pract. 2012;66(5):477–92.

Bengel MF, Higuchi T, et al. Cardiac positron emission tomography. J Am Coll Cardiol. 2009;54:1–15.

Berman DS, Hachamovitch R, Shaw LJ, et al. Roles of nuclear cardiology, cardiac computed tomography, and cardiac magnetic resonance: Noninvasive risk stratification and a conceptual framework for the selection of noninvasive imaging tests in patients with known or suspected coronary artery disease. J Nucl Med. 2006;47:1107.

Bonow RO, Mann LD, Zipes PD, et al. Braunwald's heart disease – a textbook of cardiovascular medicine. 9th ed. Philadelphia, PA: Elsevier Saunders; 2011.

Brindis RG, Douglas PS, Hendel RC, et al. ACCF/ASNC appropriateness criteria for single-photon emission computed tomography myocardial perfusion imaging (SPECT MPI): A report of the American College of Cardiology Foundation Quality Strategic Directions Committee Appropriateness Criteria Working Group and the American Society of Nuclear Cardiology endorsed by the American Heart Association. J Am Coll Cardiol. 2005;46:1587.

Burrell S, MacDonald A. Artifacts and pitfalls in myocardial perfusion imaging. J Nucl Med Technol. 2006;34:193–211.

Cerqueira MD, Allman KC, Ficaro EP, et al. Recommendations for reducing radiation exposure in myocardial perfusion imaging. J Nucl Cardiol. 2010;17:709.

Cerqueira MD, Weissman NJ, Dilsizian V, et al. Standardized myocardial segmentation and nomenclature for tomographic imaging of the heart: A statement for healthcare professionals from the cardiac imaging committee of the council on clinical cardiology of the American Heart Association. Circulation. 2002;105:539.

Chaitman BR. Should early acceleration of heart rate during exercise be used to risk stratify patients with suspected or established coronary artery disease? Circulation. 2007;115:430.

Chamarthy M, Travin IM. Altered biodistribution and incidental findings on myocardial perfusion imaging. Semin Nucl Med. 2010;40:257–70.

Chen J, Henneman MM, Trimble MA, et al. Assessment of left ventricular mechanical dyssynchrony by phase analysis of ECG-gated SPECT myocardial perfusion imaging. J Nucl Cardiol. 2008;15:127–36.

Christian PE, Bernier DR, Langan JK. Nuclear medicine and PET. Technology and techniques. 5th ed. St. Louis, MO: Mosby; 2004.

Coakley AJ, Kettle AG, Wells CP, et al. 99mTcsestamibi: a new agent for parathyroid imaging. Nucl Med Commun. 1989;10:791–4.

Cooper JA, Neumann PH, McCandless BK. Effect of patient motion on tomographic myocardial perfusion imaging. J Nucl Med. 1992;33:1566–71.

Des Prez RD, et al. ASNC Clinical Update: stress-only myocardial perfusion imaging. J Nucl Cardiol. 2009;39:999–1004.

DePuey EG. Advances in SPECT camera software and hardware: currently available and new on the horizon. J Nucl Cardiol. 2012 Jun;19(3):551–81.

Dilsizian V, Narula J, Braunwald E, Dilsizian V, Narula J, Braunwald E, editors. Atlas of nuclear cardiology. 3rd ed. Philadelphia, PA: Current Medicine; 2009.

Dorbala S, Hachamovitch R, Curillova Z, et al. Incremental prognostic value of gated Rb-82 positron emission tomography myocardial perfusion imaging over clinical variables and rest LVEF. JACC Cardiovasc Imaging. 2009;2:846–54.

Early PJ, Sodee BD. Principles and practice of nuclear medicine. 2nd ed. St. Louis, MO: Mosby; 1995.

Fam NP, Verma S, Kutryk M, et al. Clinician guide to angiogenesis. Circulation. 2003;108: 2613–8.

Fang CJ, Aranki S. Diagnosis and management of ischemic cardiomyopathy http://www.uptodate.com/contents/diagnosis-and-management-of-ischemic-cardiomyopathy.

Ficaro EP, Hansen CL, American Society of Nuclear Cardiology: Imaging Guidelines for Nuclear Cardiology Procedures. Available at: http://www.asnc.org/imageuploads/ImagingGuidelinesComplete070709.pdf.

Ficaro EP, Kritzman JN, Corbett JR. Effect of valve plane constraint on LV ejection fractions from gated perfusion SPECT [abstract]. J Nucl Cardiol. 2003;10:S23.

Fox KAA, Birkhead J, Wilcox R, Knight C, Barth J. British Cardiac Society Working Group on the definition of myocardial infarction. Heart. 2004;90:603–9.

Froelicher VF, Myers J. Exercise and the heart. 5th ed. Philadelphia, PA: WB Saunders; 2006.

Frohlich ED. Rypin's basic sciences review. 18th ed. Philadelphia, PA: J. B. Lippincott Company; 2001.

Fuster V, O'Rourke RA, Walsh RA, Poole WP. Hurst's the heart. 12th ed. New York: McGraw Hill; 2007.

Germano G. Technical aspects of myocardial SPECT imaging. J Nucl Med. 2001;42:1499–507.

Germano G, Berman SD. Clinical gated cardiac SPECT. 2nd ed. Malden, MA: Blackwell Publishing; 2006.

Gheorghiade M, Sopko G, De Luca L, et al. Navigating the crossroads of coronary artery disease and heart failure. Circulation. 2006;114:1202.

Ghosh N, Rimoldi EO, Beanlands SBR, et al. Assessment of myocardial ischaemia and viability: role of positron emission tomography. Eur Heart J. 2010;31:2984–95.

Gibbons JR. Imaging techniques. Myocardial perfusion imaging. Heart. 2000;83:355–60.

Goldberger LA. Clinical electrocardiography: a simplified approach. 7th ed. St. Louis, MO: Mosby Elsevier; 2006.

Goldman L, Schafer IA, editors. Goldman: Goldman's Cecil medicine. 24th ed. Philadelphia, PA: Saunders, an imprint of Elsevier; 2012.

Heller VG, Hendel CR. Nuclear cardiology: practical applications. 2nd ed. New York: McGraw-Hill; 2011.

Heller VG, Lundbye BJ, Kapetanopoulos A. Vasodilator stress radionuclide myocardial perfusion imaging: testing methodologies and safety. http://www.uptodate.com

Hendel CR, et al. ACCF/ASNC/ACR/AHA/ASE/SCCT/SCMR/SNM 2009 Appropriate use criteria for cardiac radionuclide imaging. J Am Coll Cardiol. 2009;53(23):2201–29.

Hill J, Timmis A. ABC of clinical electrocardiography. Exercise tolerance testing. http://www.ncbi.nlm.nih.gov/pmc/articles/PMC1123032/pdf/1084.pdf.

Ho BV, Reddy PG. Cardiovascular imaging. 1st ed. St. Louis, Mo: Saunders; 2011.

Holly AT, Abbott GB, Al-Mallah M, et al. ASNC imaging guidelines for nuclear cardiology procedures. Single photon-emission computed tomography. J Nucl Cardiol. 2010;17:1071–3581.

Husain SS. Myocardial perfusion imaging protocols: is there an ideal protocol? J Nucl Med Technol. 2007;35:3–9.

ICRP 1991 The 1990 recommendations of the International Commission on Radiological Protection. ICRP Publication 60. Ann ICRP21. Pergamon, Oxford.

Iskandar A et al. Gender differences in the diagnostic accuracy of SPECT myocardial perfusion imaging: a bivariate meta-analysis. ASNC 2012

Iskandrian EA, Garcia VE. Atlas of nuclear cardiology: imaging companion to Braunwald's heart disease. Philadelphia, PA: Elsevier Saunders; 2012.

Iskandrian AE, Verani MS, et al. Nuclear cardiac imaging and principles applications. 3rd ed. New York: Oxford University Press; 2003.

Khalil MM, editor. Basic sciences of nuclear medicine. Berlin: Springer; 2011.

Kinahan PE, Townsend DW, Beyer T, et al. Attenuation correction for a combined 3D PET/CT scanner. Med Phys. 1998;25:2046–53.

Klabunde ER. Cardiovascular physiology concepts. http://www.cvphysiology.com/CAD/CAD003.htm

Koller D. Assessing diagnostic performance in nuclear cardiology. J Nucl Cardiol. 2002;9:114–23.

Kumar V, et al. Robbins & Cotran pathologic basis of disease. 8th ed. Philadelphia, PA: Saunders; 2009.

Lauer SM. Heart rate response in stress testing: clinical implications. ACC CURRENT JOURNAL REVIEW Sep/Oct 2001.

Lenneman A, Ooi HH et al. Cardiogenic shock. http://emedicine.medscape.com/article/152191-overview. Accessed May 21 2012.

Lin CE, Alavi A. PET and PET/CT. A clinical guide. 2nd ed. New York, NY: Thieme; 2009.

Lombardi MH. Radiation safety in nuclear medicine. Boca Raton, FL: CRC Press LLC; 1999.

Lu E, Wagner WR, Schellenberger U, et al. Targeted in vivo labeling of receptors for vascular endothelial growth factor: approach to identification of ischemic tissue. Circulation. 2003;108:97–103.

Manglos SH, Thomas FD, Gagne GM, Hellwig BJ. Phantom study of breast tissue attenuation in myocardial imaging. J Nucl Med. 1993;34:992.

MacDonald A, Burrell AS. Infrequently performed studies in nuclear medicine: part 1. J Nucl Med Technol. 2008;36:132–43.

Mark DB, Hlatky MA, Harrell Jr FE, Lee KL, Califf RM, Pryor DB. Exercise treadmill score for predicting prognosis in coronary artery disease. Ann Intern Med. 1987;106:793–800.

Miyamoto IM, Vernotico LS, Majmundar H, Thomas SG. Pharmacologic stress myocardial perfusion imaging: A practical approach. J Nucl Cardiol. 2007;14:250–5.

Morrison RA, Sinusas JA. New molecular imaging targets to characterize myocardial biology. Cardiol Clin. 2009;27:329–44.

Papaioannou IG, Heller VG. Exercise radionuclide myocardial perfusion imaging in the diagnosis and prognosis of coronary heart disease. http://www.uptodate.com

Parker RP, Smith PHS, Taylor DM. Basic science of nuclear medicine. 2nd ed. Edinburgh: Churchill Livingstone; 1984.

Paul KI, Nabi AH. Gated myocardial perfusion SPECT: basic principles, technical aspects, and clinical applications. J Nucl Med Technol. 2004;32:179–87.

Pharmacotherapeutics. http://www.uic.edu/classes/pmpr/pmpr652/Final/bressler/chemocardiac.html.

Pichler BJ, Wehrl HF, Judenhofer MS. Latest advances in molecular imaging instrumentation. J Nucl Med. 2008;49 Suppl 2:5S–23S.

Rahmima A, Zaidib HA. PET versus SPECT: strengths, limitations and challenges. Nucl Med Commun. 2008;29(3):193–207.

Saladin SK. Anatomy and physiology: the unity of form and function. 5th ed. New York: McGraw-Hill Higher Education; 2009.

Scanlon PJ, Faxon DP, Audet AM, et al. ACC/AHA guidelines for coronary angiography. A report of the American College of Cardiology/American Heart Association Task Force on practice guidelines. J Am Coll Cardiol. 1999;33:1756–824.

Schelbert RH. Quantification of myocardial blood flow: what is the clinical Role? Cardiol Clin. 2009;27:277–89.

Schinkel FLA, Poldermans D, Elhendy A, Bax JJ. Assessment of myocardial viability in patients with heart failure. J Nucl Med. 2007;48:1135–46.

Schlosser T, Pagonidis K, Herborn UC, et al. Assessment of left ventricular parameters using 16-MDCT: results. Am J Roentgenol. 2005;184(3):765–73.

Sica TG. Bias in research studies. Radiology. Vol.238 (3), 2006

The Society of Nuclear Medicine, the American Heart Association, the American College of Cardiology. Standardization of cardiac tomographic imaging. J Nucl Med. 1992;33(7): 1434–5.

Statkiewicz-Sherer MA, Ritenour ER, Visconti PJ. Radiation protection in medical radiography. 6th ed. Maryland Heights, MO: Mosby; 2011.

Strauss WH, Grewal KR, Pandit-Taskar N. Molecular imaging in nuclear cardiology. Semin. 2004;XXXIV(1):47–55.

Strickberger SA, et al. AHA/ACCF scientific statement on the evaluation of syncope. Circulation. 2006;113:316–27.

Takalkar A, Agarwal A, Adams S, et al. Cardiac Assessment with PET. PET Clin. 2011;6:313–26.

Takalkar A, ChenW, Desjardins B et al. Cardiovascular imaging with PET CT and MR imaging. PET Clin 2008; 3(3)

Thompson K, Saab G, Birnie D, Chow BJ, et al. Is septal glucose metabolism altered in patients with left bundle branch block and ischemic cardiomyopathy? J Nucl Med. 2006;47:1763–8.

Treves ST, Blume ED, Armsby L, Newburger JW, Kurac A. Cardiovascular system. In: Treves ST, editor. Pediatric nuclear medicine/PET. 3rd ed. New York, NY: Springer; 2007. p. 128–61.

Van Train KF, Garcia EV, Maddahi J, et al. Multicenter trial validation for quantitative analysis of same-day rest-stress technetium-99m-sestamibi myocardial tomograms. J Nucl Med. 1994;35:609–18.

Weiner AD. Stress testing to determine prognosis and management of patients with known or suspected coronary heart disease. http://www.uptodate.com.

Weissleder R, Wittenberg J, Harisinghani GM, Chen WJ. Primer of diagnostic imaging. 5th ed. St. Louis, MO: Elsevier Mosby; 2011.

Wheat J, Currie G. Incidence and characterisation of patient motion in myocardial perfusion SPECT imaging: part 1. J Nucl Med Technol. 2004;32(2):60–5.

Zaidi H, Hasegawa B. Determination of the attenuation map in emission tomography. J Nucl Med. 2003;44:291.

Zaret BL, Beller GA. Clinical nuclear cardiology: state of the art and future directions. 3rd ed. Philadelphia, PA: Mosby; 2005.

Zubal GI, Wisniewski G. Understanding Fourier space and filter selection. J Nucl Cardiol. 1997;4:234–43.

Chapter 4
Practice Test #3: Difficulty Level—Hard

Andrzej Moniuszko and B. Adrian Kesala

Questions

1. All of the following features discovered on stress SPECT MPI identify patients with high risk (>3 % annual mortality rate) EXCEPT:
   A. Stress induced large perfusion defect
   B. Large, fixed perfusion defect with left ventricular dilatation
   C. Post-stress ejection fraction >35 %
   D. Stress induced multiple perfusion defects of moderate size

2. A recognized phenomenon in myocardial perfusion SPECT, often attributed to reduced myocardial width at the tip of the left ventricle, is called:
   A. Apical thinning
   B. Diaphragm attenuation
   C. Liver attenuation
   D. Upward creep

3. The visualization of abnormalities, provoked by ischemia and sustained even after restoration of perfusion is called:
   A. Coronary artery calcium imaging
   B. Functional imaging
   C. Myocardial ischemic memory imaging
   D. Viability imaging

Answers to Test #3 begin on page 198

A. Moniuszko, ARRT (N), PET, NCT. (✉) • B.A. Kesala, M.D.
Department of Radiology, Staff Radiologist, Presence Resurrection Medical Center,
7435 West Talcott Avenue, Chicago, Cook County, IL 60631, USA
e-mail: mdandy52@yahoo.com

A. Moniuszko and B.A. Kesala, *Nuclear Cardiology Study Guide: A Technologist's Review for Passing Specialty Certification Exams*, DOI 10.1007/978-1-4614-8645-9_4, © Springer Science+Business Media New York 2014

4. Respiratory and contractile cardiac motion during a CT portion of hybrid imaging:
   A. Markedly impacts the attenuation correction when compared with a transmission scan
   B. Has no effect on the attenuation correction
   C. Is temporally averaged
   D. Impacts the attenuation correction to a degree comparable with a transmission scan

5. The subendocardium is more susceptible to myocardial ischemia than the subepicardium because of:
   A. Decreased wall contractility
   B. Decreased wall motion
   C. Increased wall tension
   D. Increased wall thickness

6. Which of the following statements correctly describes the diagnostic role of gating in myocardial perfusion SPECT?
   A. GSPECT yields more abnormal segments in comparison with perfusion alone
   B. Gating increases the reader's confidence in interpretation of the perfusion scan
   C. GSPECT helps classify a fixed perfusion defect as a soft-tissue attenuation artifact or an infarct
   D. Gating doesn't help to differentiate ischemic from nonischemic, dilated cardiomyopathy

7. Peak pharmacological effects of dipyridamole, following initiation of infusion, occur at:
   A. About 1–2 min
   B. About 2–4 min
   C. About 4–6 min
   D. About 6–8 min

8. A mathematical statement describing the relationships of test sensitivity, specificity, and the predictive value of a positive test result is called:
   A. Bayes' theorem
   B. Fourier transform
   C. Mortality
   D. Prevalence

9. A major source of error in SPECT reconstruction is data filtering; applying filters that are too smooth may result in an increase of:
   A. False positive studies
   B. True positive studies
   C. False negative studies
   D. False positive studies

10. Anticipation of dynamic exercise results in all of the following EXCEPT:
    A. An acceleration of ventricular rate
    B. Increased venous return
    C. Increase in alveolar ventilation
    D. Increased muscle oxygen extraction

11. Which of the following tracers has ~50 % myocardial clearance at 10 min?
    A. Tc-99m sestamibi
    B. Tc-99m teboroxime
    C. Tc-99m tetrofosmin
    D. Thallium-201

12. The mathematical domain within which images can be described through the use of "spatial frequencies," is called:
    A. Fourier transform
    B. Fourier space
    C. Radon space
    D. Radon transform

13. The normal variant in myocardial perfusion images known as the "drop-out of the upper septum," is related to:
    A. Structural variations of the myocardium—the apex is anatomically thinner than other myocardial regions
    B. Structural variations of the myocardium—the muscular septum is merging with the membranous septum
    C. Technical factors—the camera is physically closer to the septal myocardial wall
    D. Technical factors—the patient motion

14. Which of the following is NOT a common cause of improper registration between the transmission and emission scans during cardiac PET/CT acquisition?
    A. Breathing motion
    B. Drift of the contents of thoracic cavity
    C. Drift of the contents of abdominal cavity
    D. Patient motion

15. Which of the following is considered the concluding proof of myocardial viability after revascularization?
    A. Improvement in exercise capacity
    B. Improvement in function
    C. Improvement in symptoms
    D. Prevention of sudden death

16. A theoretical point during dynamic exercise when muscle tissue switches over to metabolism without oxygen is called:
    A. Aerobic metabolism
    B. Aerobic threshold
    C. Anaerobic metabolism
    D. Anaerobic threshold

17. The timing of the appearance of radiation-induced leukemia is about:
    A. 1 year postirradiation
    B. 3 years postirradiation
    C. 7 years postirradiation
    D. 14 years postirradiation

18. According to recommendations from the U.S. Preventive Services Task Force (USPSTF), which population of asymptomatic adults should generally receive screening for coronary heart disease with resting or exercise electrocardiography (ECG)?
    A. Low risk
    B. Intermediate risk
    C. High risk
    D. None of the above

19. Persistent LV dysfunction on poststress GSPECT indicates:
    A. Increased exercise capabilities
    B. A high-grade coronary stenosis
    C. A low grade stenosis
    D. Radiotracer intolerance

20. The Borg scale is used to estimate:
    A. Anaerobic threshold
    B. Treadmill speed
    C. Perceived patient exertion
    D. Maximal heart rate

21. The sensitivity of pharmacologic stress is considered to be equal to that of an exercise stress test in which:
    A. The maximal 55 % of age-predicted heart rate is reached
    B. The maximal 65 % of age-predicted heart rate is reached
    C. The maximal 75 % of age-predicted heart rate is reached
    D. The maximal 85 % of age-predicted heart rate is reached

22. The method by which a recognizable image is constructed—summing spatial frequencies—is called:
    A. Fourier transform
    B. Fourier space
    C. Inverse Fourier transform
    D. Fourier rebinning

23. The conversion of the CT image into an attenuation map in which the attenuation coefficients are assessed by multiplying the CT numbers by the ratio of the water attenuation coefficients at the SPECT and CT energies is called:
    A. Scaling method
    B. Segmentation method
    C. Hybrid technique
    D. Projection technique

24. For the 511-keV photons, soft tissue attenuation per centimeter:
    A. Is not affected by the type of tissue
    B. Is less than the attenuation of the 80- to 140-keV photons emitted by SPECT radiotracers
    C. Is more than the attenuation of the 80- to 140-keV photons emitted by SPECT radiotracers
    D. Is the same as the attenuation of 80- to 140-keV photons emitted by SPECT radiotracers

25. An absolute decrease in flow, distal to a coronary stenosis, in response to coronary vasodilation occurring within the coronary artery territory (endocardial to epicardial), is called:
    A. Flow reserve
    B. Intracoronary steal
    C. Intercoronary steal
    D. Reverse flow

26. All of the following approaches have been used to correct attenuation artifacts in SPECT cardiac imaging EXCEPT:
    A. An "interleaved" attenuation correction
    B. A sequential attenuation correction
    C. A simultaneous attenuation correction
    D. A simulated attenuation correction

27. A 63-year-old man with history of CABG presents to ED with complaints of intermittent lightheadedness and dizziness. He has type 2 diabetes and is hypertensive. His ECG (Fig. 4.1) shows the presence of an implantable:
    A. Atrial pacemaker
    B. Biventricular pacemaker
    C. Cardioverter-defibrillator
    D. Ventricular pacemaker

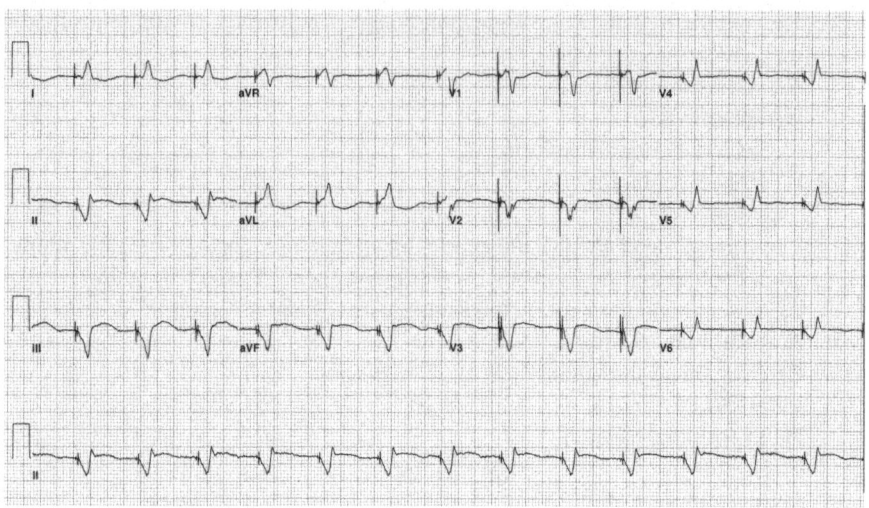

Fig. 4.1 Electrocardiogram

28. I-131 labeled monocyte chemoattractant protein 1 has been shown to accumulate in lipid-rich, macrophage-rich regions in animal models of:
    A. Angiogenesis
    B. Arrhythmia
    C. Atherosclerosis
    D. Cancer

29. According to the ASNC recommendations, by 2014, a goal is set to decrease patient radiation exposure associated with myocardial perfusion imaging SPECT to less than:
    A. 18 mSv in 100 % of patients
    B. 18 mSv in 50 % of patients
    C. 9 mSv in 100 % of patients
    D. 9 mSv in 50 % of patients

30. The only significant mechanism available to the heart to increase oxygen consumption is to:
    A. Increase oxygen extraction
    B. Increase fatty acids consumption
    C. Increase perfusion
    D. Increase glucose utilization

31. The American Society of Nuclear Cardiology and the Society of Nuclear Medicine together recommend:
    A. Against applying attenuation correction in addition to ECG gating with SPECT MPI
    B. In favor of applying attenuation correction in addition to ECG gating with SPECT MPI
    C. Against applying attenuation correction without ECG gating with SPECT MPI
    D. In favor of applying attenuation correction without ECG gating with SPECT MPI

32. Peripheral sites, other than the antecubital (preferably medial) and external jugular veins, are NOT suitable for first-pass radionuclide angiography (FPRNA) because of the possibility of bolus (select two):
    A. Extravasation
    B. Fractionation
    C. Infiltration
    D. Prolongation
    E. Reduction

33. Automated method that adjusts the intensity of the myocardial perfusion image to reflect the estimated magnitude of soft tissue tempering on different regions of the heart is called:
    A. Filtering
    B. Attenuation correction
    C. Image fusion
    D. Smoothing

34. During PET/CT acquisition:
    A. PET emission data and CT scanner "freeze" the heart, lungs, and liver at one point in the respiratory cycle
    B. PET emission data "freeze" the heart, lungs, and liver at one point in the respiratory cycle, whereas the CT scanner averages many respiratory cycles
    C. CT scanner "freezes" the heart, lungs, and liver at one point in the respiratory cycle, whereas the PET emission data are averaged over many respiratory cycles
    D. CT scanner and the PET emission data are averaged over many respiratory cycles

35. When the existence of a cardiac shunt is assessed using the first pass technique, reappearance of activity in the lungs shortly after the first pass, but before recirculation through body:
    A. Indicates the presence of R–L shunt
    B. Excludes the presence of R–L shunt
    C. Indicates the presence of L–R shunt
    D. Excludes the presence of L–R shunt

36. An event that can be demonstrated, using sequential exercise testing, when the time to angina and ischemic ST-segment depression can be prolonged on the second of two exercise tests, is known as:
    A. Adaptive response
    B. ST normalization
    C. T wave pseudonormalization
    D. Warm-up phenomenon

37. The unit of cut-off frequency is:
    A. cm
    B. cm^2
    C. cm^{-1}
    D. cm^3

38. The Fick Principle describes the relationship between myocardial oxygen consumption or mixed venous oxygen saturation (MVO$_2$), coronary blood flow (CBF), and the:
    A. Arterial-venous oxygen difference
    B. Glucose level
    C. Heart rate
    D. Level of exercise

39. The biological half-life of Tl-201 is approximately:
    A. 1 day
    B. 5 days
    C. 10 days
    D. 20 days

40. Perceived exertion ratings between 12 and 14 on the Borg Scale suggest that physical activity is being performed at a:
    A. Very light level
    B. Light level of intensity
    C. Moderate level of intensity
    D. Very hard level of intensity

41. Which of the following statements describing motion artifacts is FALSE?
    A. The number of frames with motion determines the magnitude of image artifact
    B. The direction and pattern of motion determine the location of artifacts
    C. Motion that occurs when the heart is close to the detector is less likely to create image artifacts
    D. The direction of motion may be lateral, vertical, or rotational

42. Activation of A1 adenosine receptors produces:
    A. Atrioventricular conduction delay
    B. Bronchospasm
    C. Coronary vasodilatation
    D. Tachycardia

43. The view comprising long-axis tomograms, generated by slicing along the horizontal plane through the short-axis perspective, is called:
    A. Vertical short-axis view
    B. Horizontal short-axis view
    C. Vertical long-axis view
    D. Horizontal long-axis view

44. The chemical form of rubidium 82 obtained from a Cardiogen-82 generator is:
    A. Rb-82 carbonate
    B. Rb-82 chloride
    C. Rb-82 oxide
    D. Rb-82 sulfur

45. The contrast echocardiography viability studies with high-molecular weight inert gases are based on evaluation of:
    A. Cell membrane integrity
    B. Contractile reserve
    C. Myocardial perfusion
    D. Scar tissue

46. Prone imaging may occasionally create a fixed defect located:
    A. Anteriorly or posteriorly
    B. Anteriorly or laterally
    C. Posteriorly or inferiorly
    D. Laterally or inferiorly

47. Which of the following statements describing the regadenoson plasma concentration-time profile is CORRECT?
    A. The maximal plasma concentration of regadenoson is within 1 min after injection of Lexiscan
    B. The half-life of initial phase is approximately 4–8 min
    C. The half-life of intermediate phase is on average 1 h
    D. The half-life of terminal phase is approximately 2 h

48. The auto-regulatory mechanism of the heart seeks to balance the supply and demand of:
    A. Amino acids
    B. Fatty acids
    C. Glucose
    D. Oxygen

49. Cadmium Zinc Telluride (CZT) crystals absorb the γ-ray energy and generate electron–hole pairs with resulting conversion of the photons into:
    A. A digital image
    B. A digital signal
    C. An electronic signal
    D. A hard copy

50. Which of the following results of the Duke Treadmill Scores (DTS) identifies patient with high risk CAD?
    A. ≤−11
    B. +4 to −10
    C. + 5 to +10
    D. ≥ +10

51. After the initial uptake and distribution of thallium, the subsequent redistribution of thallium begins within:
    A. 5–10 min after injection
    B. 10–15 min after injection
    C. 15–20 min after injection
    D. 20–25 min after injection

52. According to the ASNC imaging guidelines, the radionuclide of choice for standard first-pass radionuclide angiography (FPRNA) is:
    A. Tc-99m sestamibi
    B. Tc-99m pertechnetate
    C. Tc-99m diethylamine triamine pentaacetic acid
    D. Tc-99m sulfur colloid

53. "Evolution" by GE Healthcare, "Astonish" by Philips, and Flash 3D by Siemens are examples of:
    A. Attenuation correction systems
    B. Hybrid systems
    C. Advanced image reconstruction techniques
    D. New camera designs

54. The PET potential for quantifying myocardial blood flow and blood flow reserve in absolute terms is highly beneficial in patients with:
    A. Balanced ischemia
    B. Myocardial infarction
    C. Hibernating myocardium
    D. Unstable angina

55. MRI and echocardiography viability studies with dobutamine are based on the evaluation of:
    A. Cell membrane integrity
    B. Contractile reserve
    C. Myocardial perfusion
    D. Scar tissue

56. Which of the following statements describing the scanning sealed source system used for the attenuation map creation in transmission computed tomography (TCT) is FALSE:
    A. The system requires strict quality control to ensure precise movement of the line source
    B. The flux of X-ray photons from a conventional sealed source is much higher than typical X-ray tube
    C. The scanning line source system is geometrically complex and less sensitive than CT-based techniques
    D. The system requires an electronic window as well as source strength

57. According to the Lexiscan package insert, nursing women may consider interrupting nursing after regadenoson administration for:
    A. 1 h
    B. 10 h
    C. 24 h
    D. 48 h

58. Research bias, introduced when there is a sufficient time delay between the application of the test, and the reference standard to allow change in the disease state, is called:
    A. Differential verification bias
    B. Disease progression bias
    C. Incorporation bias
    D. Treatment paradox bias

59. In patients with a normal MPI study, the hard event rate (cardiac death or non-fatal myocardial infarction) occurring during an average follow-up of 2 years is approximately:
    A. 0.7 % per year
    B. 1.4 % per year
    C. 2.3 % per year
    D. 3.0 % per year

60. A deceleration of heart rate following exercise termination is called:
    A. Chronotropic incompetence
    B. Inotropic incompetence
    C. Heart rate recovery
    D. Sinus bradycardia

61. The transmission-to-cross-talk ratio (TCR) depends on all of the following
    EXCEPT:
    A. The injected activity
    B. The transmission source strength
    C. The body habitus
    D. The camera sensitivity

62. Which of the following adenosine receptors stimulation may result in bron-
    chial constriction and peripheral vasodilation?
    A. A1
    B. A2a
    C. A2b
    D. A3

63. According to the appropriate use criteria (AUC), which of the following tests
    will be appropriate for an exercising regularly 54-year-old woman presented
    with atypical chest pain, hx of hypertension, hypercholesterolemia, and sec-
    ondary to LVH resting ECG changes?
    A. Cardiac CT
    B. Coronary angiogram
    C. Exercise ECG
    D. Stress radionuclide MPI

64. The PET perfusion imaging agents: F-18-fluorobenzyl triphenyl phospho-
    nium and F-18 flupiridaz bind to the:
    A. Cell wall
    B. Lysosome
    C. Mitochondria
    D. Nuclear membrane

65. All of the following response patterns can be observed on echocardiography
    viability studies with low dose dobutamine infusion EXCEPT:
    A. Biphasic response
    B. Sustained improvement
    C. Triphasic response
    D. Worsening

66. Patients with inferior wall abnormalities on supine imaging, that were absent
    on prone imaging, had a risk of subsequent cardiac events that is comparable
    to the risk in patients with:
    A. Summed stress score more than 25 on supine-only studies
    B. Summed stress score more than 15 on supine-only studies
    C. Summed stress score more than 5 on supine-only studies
    D. Normal supine-only studies

67. Adenosine produces vasoconstriction in:
    A. Coronary arteries
    B. Coronary veins
    C. Renal afferent arterioles
    D. Pulmonary veins

68. In patients with coronary artery disease, coronary flow reserve decreases in proportion to the degree of stenosis severity and is exhausted for stenosis:
    A. $\geq 20\,\%$
    B. $\geq 40\,\%$
    C. $\geq 60\,\%$
    D. $\geq 80\,\%$

69. Which of the following is the energy supplier for the cell?
    A. Lysosome
    B. Mitochondria
    C. Ribosome
    D. Vacuole

70. All of the following baseline electrocardiographic abnormalities may preclude use of exercise ECG for noninvasive stress testing EXCEPT:
    A. Left bundle branch block
    B. Premature atrial contractions
    C. Permanent ventricular pacing
    D. Ventricular pre-excitation syndrome

71. High-speed SPECT technology introduces a series of small, pixilated solid-state detector columns equipped with:
    A. NaTI crystals
    B. LYSO crystals
    C. CsI(Tl) crystals
    D. BGO crystals

72. After an intravenous injection of Tc 99m macroaggregated albumin, an increased portion of perfusion getting into systemic circulation rather than the lungs is referred to as:
    A. Pulmonary hypertension
    B. The percentage R–L shunt
    C. The percentage L–R shunt
    D. Pulmonary embolism

73. A 79-year-old man presents to ED with complaints of intermittent lighthead-
    edness and dizziness. He has type 2 diabetes and is hypertensive. What are the
    ECG (Fig. 4.2) findings?
    A. Atrial fibrillation with rapid ventricular response
    B. Atrial flutter with variable A–V block
    C. Sinus rhythm with frequent PVCs in a pattern of bigeminy
    D. Sinus tachycardia with frequent PACs

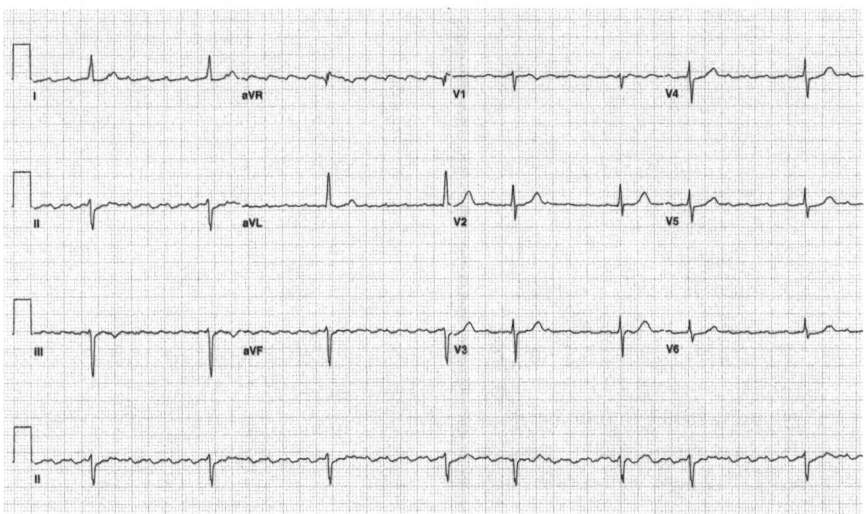

Fig. 4.2 Electrocardiogram

74. F-18 fluorodexyglucose is transported into the myocyte by the sarcolemmal
    glucose transporters:
    A. GLUT 3 and GLUT 6
    B. GLUT 2 and GLUT 5
    C. GLUT1 and GLUT 4
    D. GLUT 0 and GLUT 3

75. The mechanism responsible for a normal MPI study, despite established CAD,
    involves preserved:
    A. Collagen fibers
    B. Endothelial function
    C. Smooth muscle
    D. Striated muscle

76. Stress ECG-gated myocardial SPECT imaging with Tc-99m-labeled agents soon after exercise is superior to conventional late imaging in identifying patients with myocardial:
    A. Infarction
    B. Inflammation
    C. Ischemia
    D. Stunning

77. The ramp filter suppresses the star artifact by controlling:
    A. High frequencies
    B. Low frequencies
    C. Medium frequencies
    D. Noise

78. Which of the following is currently considered as the gold standard for ventricular volumes and function measurements?
    A. GSPECT
    B. ECHO
    C. MRI
    D. MUGA

79. Which of the following statements describing radionuclide angiography (RNA) is FALSE?
    A. RNA can be performed with each a planar technique or tomography
    B. RNA can be done at rest or with exercise
    C. RNA-derived EF is based on geometric assumptions
    D. RNA can be completed with first-pass and gated equilibrium approaches

80. The pulmonary vascular bed can accommodate as much as a/an _____ increase in cardiac output.
    A. Twofold
    B. Fourfold
    C. Sixfold
    D. Eightfold

81. The highest spatial frequency that can be encoded in the digital image is called:
    A. Temporal
    B. Nyquist
    C. Fourier
    D. Limited

82. Administration of dipyridamole, adenosine, or regadenoson results in:
    A. An 8–10 mm Hg increase in systolic and diastolic blood pressure and reflex increase in heart rate by 10 and 20 beats/min
    B. A reduction of 8–10 mm Hg in systolic and diastolic blood pressure and reflex increase in heart rate by 10 and 20 beats/min
    C. A reduction of 8–10 mm Hg in systolic and diastolic blood pressure and reflex decrease in heart rate by 10 and 20 beats/min
    D. An 8–10 mm Hg increase in systolic and diastolic blood pressure and reflex decrease in heart rate by 10 and 20 beats/min

83. Which of the following LV function parameters is assessed by evaluating the changes in brightness from the end-diastolic to the end-systolic frame?
    A. Regional wall motion
    B. Systolic wall thickening
    C. Regional EF
    D. Global EF

84. During the cardiac PET/CT acquisition, the respiratory cycle can be monitored by using all of the following EXCEPT:
    A. A bellows
    B. A chest band
    C. An electrocardiograph
    D. An infrared tracking system

85. According to the American College of Cardiology guidelines, patients with a 75 % pretest likelihood of CAD are considered to be:
    A. Not at risk for CAD
    B. At low risk for CAD
    C. At moderate risk for CAD
    D. At high risk of CAD

86. Which of the following statements describing the radiation safety approach in breast-feeding mothers referred for radionuclide imaging is INCORRECT?
    A. The breasts can be pumped before the injection of radioisotope and the milk can be stored in
    B. The refrigerator for 5 days
    C. The breasts can be pumped before the injection of radioisotope and the milk can be frozen for up to 6 month.
    D. After the injection of the radioisotope, the milk can be collected and after allowing appropriate decay can be given to the infant
    E. After the injection of the radioisotope, the milk can be collected and given to the infant

87. Adenosine is a naturally occurring purine nucleoside that forms from the breakdown of:
    A. Adenosine monophosphate (AMP)
    B. Adenosine diphosphate (ADP)
    C. Adenosine triphosphate (ATP)
    D. Cyclic guanosine monophosphate (cGMP)

88. A phenomenon when dilation of one vascular network "redirects" blood flow from another region within the organ that is already maximally dilated, because of the presence of proximal lesions, is called the coronary:
    A. Collaterals
    B. Steal
    C. Fistula
    D. Atherosclerosis

89. I-123 mIBG imaging produces a quantitative index called:
    A. Ejection fraction
    B. Heart-to-mediastinum ratio
    C. Lung uptake index
    D. Transient ischemic dilation

90. Which of the following is the strongest and most consistent prognostic marker identified in exercise testing?
    A. Chest pain
    B. J point depression
    C. Maximum exercise capacity
    D. Premature atrial contractions

91. Soft tissue attenuation from breasts may produce MPI artifacts in up to:
    A. 20 % studies in women
    B. 40 % studies in women
    C. 60% studies in women
    D. 80% studies in women

92. When performing the first pass study, the integrity of the bolus is assessed by placing a ROI over the:
    A. Inferior vena cava
    B. Right atrium
    C. Right ventricle
    D. Superior vena cava

93. When cardiac death and nonfatal myocardial infarction are considered as separate endpoints, functional and perfusion data obtained from GSPECT suggests:
    A. Post-stress LVEF is the best predictor of nonfatal infarction, whereas the amount of ischemia is the best predictor of cardiac death
    B. Post-stress LVEF is the best predictor of cardiac death, whereas the amount of ischemia is the best predictor of nonfatal infarction
    C. Post-stress LVEF and the amount of ischemia are the best predictors of nonfatal infarction
    D. Post-stress LVEF and the amount of ischemia are the best predictors of cardiac death

94. An iterative reconstruction begins with:
    A. Scatter correction
    B. A guess of the image
    C. Simulate scanning
    D. Random correction

95. The hypothesis stating that accuracy of any test depends on the pretest probability of disease in the patient population being studied is known as:
    A. Bayes' theorem
    B. Fourier transform
    C. Iterative algorithm
    D. Prevalence rates

96. The adenosine infusion should be discontinued early under any of the following circumstances EXCEPT:
    A. Diastolic blood pressure >90 mm Hg
    B. Patient's request to stop
    C. Systolic blood pressure <80 mm Hg
    D. Wheezing

97. Which of the following algorithms can be used to measure LV diastolic dyssynchrony from gated SPECT MPI?
    A. Global ejection fraction
    B. Phase analysis
    C. Wall motion
    D. Wall thickening

98. The myocardium of patients with systolic heart failure is characterized by:
    A. A reduction of presynaptic norepinephrine uptake and reduction in postsynaptic β-adrenoceptor density
    B. An increase in presynaptic norepinephrine uptake and increase in postsynaptic β-adrenoceptor density
    C. An increase in presynaptic norepinephrine uptake and reduction in postsynaptic β-adrenoceptor density
    D. A reduction of presynaptic norepinephrine uptake and increase in postsynaptic β-adrenoceptor density

99. Functional improvement after coronary artery bypass grafting, or percutane-
    ous angioplasty when evaluated by GSPECT, is apparent by an/a:
    A. Increase in the ESV, a decrease in the LVEF
    B. Increase in the LVEF and in the ESV
    C. Decrease in the LVEF and in the ESV
    D. Increase in the LVEF, a decrease in the ESV

100. Perceived exertion ratings between 18 and 20 on the Borg Scale suggest that
     physical activity is being performed at:
     A. A light level of intensity
     B. A moderate level of intensity
     C. A very hard level of intensity
     D. A patient's maximum exercise capacity

101. Which of the following exercise stress test findings/symptoms indicate a high
     probability of coronary artery disease (select three)?
     A. Angina like chest pain
     B. Fall in blood pressure
     C. T wave decrease in height
     D. Substantial ST depression at low work rate
     E. Tachycardia

102. The upright over supine position for performing first-pass radionuclide angi-
     ography (FPRNA) is preferred because:
     A. Liver background is reduced in the upright position
     B. Pulmonary background is reduced in the upright position
     C. Liver background is increased in the upright position
     D. Pulmonary background is increased in the upright position

103. Which of the following variables increase sensitivity of MPI?
     A. Left circumflex coronary stenosis
     B. Branch vessel or distal stenosis
     C. Inadequate heart rate response during exercise
     D. Proximal location of stenosis

104. Rubidium acts like a microsphere that crosses the capillary membrane and is
     trapped because of:
     A. Change charge state
     B. Decay process
     C. Its size
     D. Change in shape

105. Which of the following medications should be stopped a week before tread-
     mill ECG testing?
     A. Aggrenox
     B. Digoxin
     C. Dipyridamole
     D. Warfarin

106. All of the following are advantages of using CT over the radionuclide-based
     transmission for attenuation correction of SPECT data EXCEPT:
     A. The CT image has less noise than transmission images acquired using
        radionuclide source
     B. The CT image can be acquired faster than a transmission image
     C. The CT source decays slower than a radionuclide source
     D. The CT images will not be influenced by cross-talk from the SPECT
        radionuclide

107. Figure 4.3 presents a LV volume curve derived from an 8-frame gated myocar-
     dial perfusion imaging study using 4D-MSPECT. Calculated ED of LV is
     approximately:
     A. 47 %
     B. 66 %
     C. 71 %
     D. 85 %

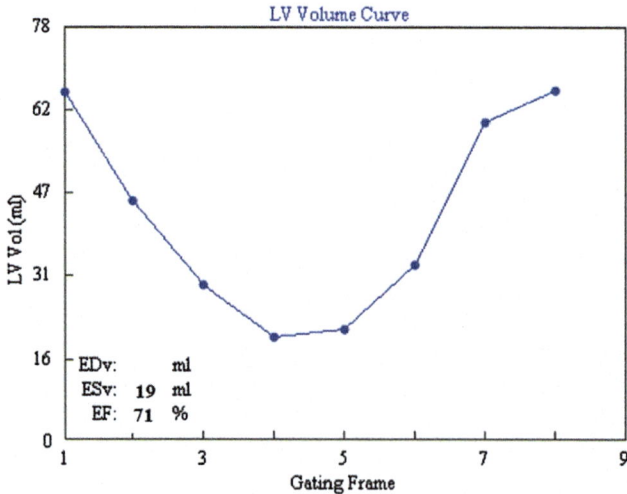

Fig. 4.3 Volume curve

108. The risk assessment tool from the Framingham Heart Study is employed to predict a person's chance of having a heart attack in the next:
    A. Year
    B. 2 years
    C. 5 years
    D. 10 years

109. Transmission imaging is a mean of creating:
    A. An emission scan
    B. An uniformity correction map
    C. An attenuation map
    D. An attenuation map

110. Cardiopulmonary exercise testing (CPET) combines exercise testing with:
    A. Blood chemistry
    B. Electrolyte analysis
    C. Myocardial perfusion imaging
    D. Ventilation gas analysis

111. The biologic half-life of dipyridamole is:
    A. 1–9 min
    B. 10–29 min
    C. 30–45 min
    D. 46–60 min

112. Which of the following radiopharmaceuticals can be used for detecting and quantifying R–L and L–R shunts?
    A. Tc-99m albumin aggregate
    B. Tc-99m sodium pertechnetate
    C. Tc-99m methylene diphosphonate
    D. Tc-99m dimercaptocuccinic acid

113. Which of the following statements comparing exercise echocardiography to exercise MPI is INCORRECT?
    A. The diagnostic accuracy of the two techniques is comparable
    B. The prognostic value of the two techniques is comparable
    C. Stress echocardiography is more accurate than stress MPI in patients with left ventricular hypertrophy
    D. Stress echocardiography is more accurate than stress MPI in patients with high body mass index

114. The two main energetic pathways used by the heart are:
    A. Amino acid and glucose metabolism
    B. Carbohydrate and fatty acid metabolism
    C. Lipid and protein metabolism
    D. Fatty acid and fructose metabolism

115. Which of the following allows dynamic assessment of cardiac function at rest and during exercise or pharmacologic agent administration?
     A. Angiography
     B. Echocardiography
     C. Electrocardiography
     D. Myocardial perfusion imaging

116. A hypertensive response to exercise is defined as one in which the systolic blood pressure rises to more than:
     A. 190 mm Hg
     B. 220 mm Hg
     C. 250 mm Hg
     D. 280 mm Hg

117. A direct negative chronotropic, dromotropic, and inotropic effect of adenosine on the heart is attributable to:
     A. The A1-receptor agonism
     B. The A1-receptor antagonism
     C. The A2-receptor agonism
     D. The A2-receptor antagonism

118. Any constellation of clinical findings that the physician feels is consistent with obstructive coronary artery disease is called:
     A. Unstable angina
     B. Ischemic equivalent
     C. Myocardial infarction
     D. Somatopsychic syndrome

119. Distance (size) in the spatial domain and frequency in the frequency domain are:
     A. Equal
     B. Proportionally related
     C. Inversely related
     D. Independent from each other

120. Which of the following is considered a relative indication to terminate an exercise stress test?
     A. Difficulties monitoring the ECG
     B. Patient request to stop the test
     C. Shortness of breath
     D. Signs of poor perfusion

121. Binodenoson and apadenoson are:
     A. Adenosine antagonists
     B. Beta blockers
     C. Calcium channel blockers
     D. Selective A2A receptor agonists

122. Radionuclide angiography (RNA) can provide information on all of the following EXCEPT:
    A. Intracardiac shunts
    B. Myocardial viability
    C. Pulmonary transit time
    D. Wall motion

123. The discordance between the times of right ventricular (RV) and left ventricular (LV) contraction is called:
    A. Diastolic incompetence
    B. Intraventricular dyssynchrony
    C. Interventricular dyssynchrony
    D. Systolic incompetence

124. The extraction of the FDG during a capillary single pass is about:
    A. 10 %
    B. 40 %
    C. 80 %
    D. 100 %

125. Which cell feature is responsible for making proteins?
    A. Lysosomes
    B. Mitochondria
    C. Ribosomes
    D. Vacuoles

126. The property of a filter that describes how quickly the transition is made between frequencies that are kept and frequencies that are eliminated is called:
    A. Cut-off
    B. Power
    C. Order
    D. Roll-on

127. With respect to its molecular structure, synaptic uptake and intracellular storage I-123 MIBG resembles the neurotransmitter:
    A. Acetylcholine
    B. Dopamine
    C. Histamine
    D. Norepinephrine

128. Which of the following occurrences is classified as a "hard event" in risk stratification in stable chest pain syndromes?
    A. Acute chest pain
    B. Heart failure
    C. Nonfatal MI
    D. Unstable angina

129. According to the current ACC/AHA guidelines for exercise testing, stopping beta-blockers before EST is discouraged to avoid:
    A. Anginal symptoms
    B. Headache
    C. Orthostatic hypotension
    D. Tachycardia

130. Specificity and sensitivity of exercise testing for the diagnosis of CAD is:
    A. 82–92 % and 74–94 % accordingly
    B. 61–73 % and 59–81 % accordingly
    C. 59–81 % and 61–73 % accordingly
    D. 74–94 % and 82–92 % accordingly

131. Inside the myocardial cell, ammonia is quickly converted to an ammonium ion, which is rapidly converted and trapped as glutamine by the enzyme:
    A. Alanine aminotransferase
    B. Aspartate aminotransferase
    C. Glutamine synthase
    D. Nitrate reductase

132. A caudal tilt of the LAO view during equilibrium radionuclide angiocardiography (ERNA) is helpful to separate:
    A. The atria from the aorta
    B. The atria from the ventricle
    C. The ventricle from the aorta
    D. The ventricles

133. Diaphragmatic attenuation is estimated to occur in up to:
    A. 5 % of myocardial perfusion studies
    B. 25 % of myocardial perfusion studies
    C. 45 % of myocardial perfusion studies
    D. 65 % of myocardial perfusion studies

134. Which of the following PET tracers has been be used to evaluate the cardiac parasympathetic nervous system?
    A. F-18 fluorodopamine
    B. F-18 fluoroethoxybenzovesamicol
    C. C-11 epinephrine
    D. C-11 phenylephrine

135. Figure 4.4 presents a screenshot of a standard LAO view MUGA scan. The arrow is pointing to the:
    A. Interatrial septum
    B. Intraatrial thrombus
    C. Interventricular septum
    D. Intraventricular thrombus

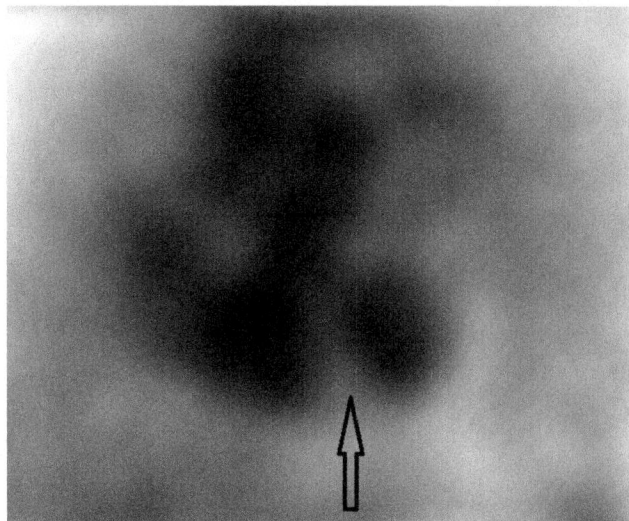

Fig. 4.4 MUGA scan

136. Which of the following baseline ECG findings DOES NOT significantly reduce the accuracy of the EST for the diagnosis of ischemia?
    A. Left bundle branch block
    B. Right bundle branch block
    C. Ventricular pacing
    D. Wolf-Parkinson-White syndrome

137. The method by which an image is transformed into its frequency components is called:
    A. Fourier transform
    B. Fourier space
    C. Inverse Fourier transform
    D. Fourier rebinning

138. The concept of "normalcy rate" has been developed in an attempt to compensate for:
    A. Age differences
    B. Gender differences
    C. Qualitative bias
    D. Referral bias

139. The absence of perfusion abnormalities in patients with dilated cardiomyopathy:
    A. Is a false negative finding
    B. Excludes CAD as the cause of the cardiomyopathy
    C. Has a low diagnostic value
    D. Indicates absence of viable myocardium

140. Low-level exercise, implemented in combination with pharmacologic stress MPI, is performed at:
    A. 0 mph, 10 % grade
    B. 1.7 mph, 0 % grade
    C. 3.5 mph, 10 %
    D. 5.0 mph, 0 % grade

141. Tc-99m sestamibi accumulates more avidly in tumor cells because tumor cells, when compared to the surrounding normal epithelial cells, have:
    A. A greater lysosomal density
    B. A greater mitochondrial density
    C. More microfilaments
    D. More ribosomes

142. The extraction phenomenon, described as a plateau of tracer uptake when myocardial blood flow is progressively increased, is called:
    A. Hibernation
    B. Stealing
    C. Roll-off
    D. Stunning

143. Which of the following statements describing extracardiac incidental findings (ECFs) on nuclear SPECT MPI is FALSE?
    A. 46 % of focal lung uptake lesions are malignant
    B. ECFs are best identified while viewing the raw data in a cine format
    C. 5 % of breast uptake lesions are malignant
    D. ECFs can be detected because of either increased or decreased tracer concentration in a ROI

144. Which of the following positron emitters can be used in centers without on-site cyclotrons?
    A. N-13 ammonia
    B. 0–15 water
    C. Palmitate C-11
    D. Rubidium-82

145. Figure 4.5 displays VLA SPECT MPI images. Label D identifies the:
    A. Anterior wall
    B. Apex
    C. Base
    D. Inferior wall

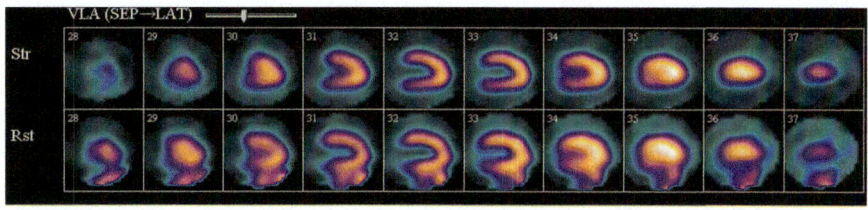

Fig. 4.5 SPECT MPI

146. Which of the following methods can be used to improve artifacts recognition in myocardial perfusion imaging (select three)?
A. ECG-gated imaging
B. Iterative algorithm
C. Prone imaging
D. Patient comforting
E. Shortened acquisition
F. Review of planar images

147. A translation formula (translation table) converts the number of acquired counts to:
A. Brightness in the image
B. Dimension of the image
C. Shape in the image
D. Sharpness of the image

148. In patients presenting with chest pain, suspected CAD, and undergoing MPI studies, the risk of cardiac death or MI increases as the:
A. Regional ejection fraction increases
B. End-systolic volume decreases
C. Number of reversible perfusion defects increases
D. Extent of inducible ischemia decreases

149. All of the following seen on stress perfusion images are the major prognostic variables predictive of future cardiac events EXCEPT:
A. Defect reversibility in multiple myocardial scan segments
B. Decreased lung Tl-201 uptake on Tl-201 scintigraphy
C. Left ventricular cavity dilation from stress to rest images
D. A resting left ventricular ejection fraction measured on Tc-99m gated SPECT imaging of <40 %

150. All of the following statements correctly describe the left ventricular function during exercise in patients with known coronary artery disease EXCEPT:
    A. EF is a reflection of the impact of regional ischemia on global LV performance
    B. Patients with three-vessel disease who have an abnormal exercise EF response are at high risk for adverse events
    C. Among patients with three-vessel disease by angiography, the EF response to exercise may be maintained
    D. Patients with three-vessel disease who have an abnormal exercise EF are less likely to benefit from revascularization

151. The use of prone imaging can reduce diaphragmatic attenuation and improve visualization of the myocardial:
    A. Posterior wall
    B. Anterior wall
    C. Septal wall
    D. Inferior wall

152. Normal wall motion and myocardial thickening in an area with a fixed defect on perfusion imaging is most likely to be classified as:
    A. An irreversible ischemia
    B. A motion artifact
    C. A reversible ischemia
    D. A soft tissue attenuation artifact

153. Which of the following statements describing efficacy of resting MPI with Tc-99m-based perfusion agents in the emergency department is FALSE?
    A. Images acquired 45–60 min later reflect myocardial blood flow at the time of injection
    B. Negative predictive value of resting MPI for ruling out myocardial infarction is high
    C. Patients with positive MPI have a higher risk of cardiac events during the index hospitalization
    D. MPI and initial troponin I values in samples drawn at the time of imaging have similar sensitivity for detection of acute MI

154. A major advantage of N-13 NH3 PET MPI, as compared with Rb-82 PET MPI, is the ability:
    A. To perform pharmaceutical stress MPI studies
    B. To perform exercise-induced stress MPI studies
    C. To perform delay imaging
    D. To acquire gated images

155. A subset of cell death that occurs as an outcome of pathologic processes outside of programmed cellular mechanisms is termed:
    A. Angiogenesis
    B. Apoptosis
    C. Arteriosclerosis
    D. Necrosis

156. The essential assumption of myocardial perfusion SPECT imaging is that the count value in each myocardial pixel (voxel) is:
    A. Directly proportional to the radiotracer concentration in the myocardium that matches that pixel
    B. Inversely proportional to the radiotracer concentration in the myocardium that matches that pixel
    C. Directly proportional to the radiotracer dose at the time of injection
    D. Inversely proportional to the radiotracer dose at the time of injection

157. Patients with normal perfusion studies at peak stress have a combined mortality and nonfatal infarction rate estimated at:
    A. <1 % per 6 months
    B. <5 % per 6 months
    C. <1 % per year
    D. <5 % per year

158. All of the following statements correctly describe efficacy of MPI when used to assess cardiac risk before noncardiac surgery EXCEPT:
    A. A normal MPI study predicts a low likelihood for perioperative cardiac events
    B. Reversible perfusion defects predict an increased risk of cardiac events
    C. Fixed perfusion defects indicate a higher risk than ischemia for perioperative cardiac events
    D. Patients with infarct or LV dysfunction are at higher long-term risk for death

159. Which of the following potential problems can be identified by reviewing a cine loop of planar rotating images (select three)?
    A. Overfiltering
    B. Soft tissue attenuation
    C. Wall motion abnormalities
    D. Abnormal lung uptake
    E. Double gating
    F. Patient motion

160. The Duke Treadmill Score (DTS) is a weighted index combining all of the following parameters EXCEPT:
    A. Maximum net ST deviation
    B. Recovery heart rate
    C. Treadmill angina index
    D. Treadmill exercise time

161. The conversion of the CT image into an attenuation map in which the CT image is allocated into regions of distinctive tissue types is called:
    A. Scaling method
    B. Segmentation method
    C. Hybrid technique
    D. Projection technique

162. An In-111 labeled quinolone (In-111RP748) demonstrates preferential binding to activated:
    A. Actins
    B. Integrins
    C. Myosins
    D. Villi

163. Which of the following statements correctly describes properties of commonly used vasodilators?
    A. Adenosine, regadenoson, and dipyridamole are equally effective in increasing coronary blood flow
    B. Dipyridamole produces slightly greater systemic vasodilation and higher peak heart rate than adenosine
    C. Adenosine offers fewer side effects, including rhythm and conduction abnormalities than regadenoson
    D. Side effects of adenosine last longer and more often require reversal with aminophylline than with dipyridamole

164. Which of the following statements correctly describes properties of Rb-82 as a myocardial perfusion tracer?
    A. Rubidium is trapped in capillaries
    B. Rubidium underestimates myocardial flow at higher rates
    C. Rubidium overestimates myocardial flow at lower rates
    D. Rubidium is a perfect microsphere analogue

165. An absolute decrease in flow, distal to a coronary stenosis in response to coronary vasodilation occurring between coronary artery territories, is called:
    A. Flow reserve
    B. Intercoronary steal
    C. Intracoronary steal
    D. Redistribution flow

166. Which of the following radiotracers can be used to image adrenergic receptors in the heart?
    A. F-18 FDG
    B. I-123 mIBG
    C. In-111 DTPA
    D. Sm-153 EDTMP

167. All of the following variables increase sensitivity of MPI EXCEPT:
    A. Antianginal therapy with nitrates
    B. High-grade coronary stenosis
    C. Presence of wall motion abnormalities
    D. Proximal location of stenosis

168. Tc-99m-labeled annexin V localizes in:
    A. Apoptotic cells
    B. Blood cells
    C. Cancer cells
    D. Inflammatory cells

169. The location of motion-induced perfusion defects-artifacts is determined by the:
    A. Magnitude of motion
    B. Timing of motion
    C. Direction of motion
    D. Number of detectors

170. A treadmill speed of 1.7 mph and a grade of 10° in a standard maximal exercise treadmill protocol is designed to achieve a workload of:
    A. 1 MET
    B. 2.3 METs
    C. 4.6 METs
    D. 8 METs

171. The intensity of the RV uptake on perfusion images is approximately:
    A. 10 % of peak LV intensity
    B. 50 % of peak LV intensity
    C. 75 % of peak LV intensity
    D. 100 % of peak LV intensity

172. Which of the following parameters by myocardial perfusion gated SPECT DOESN'T describe diastolic function?
    A. Myocardial thickening
    B. Peak to filling rate
    C. Time to peak filling rate
    D. The mean filling fraction

173. A 91-year-old woman presents to ED with increasing shortness of breath and dizziness. She has type 2 diabetes and is hypertensive. Her ECG (Fig. 4.6) shows:
    A. Atrial fibrillation with rapid ventricular response
    B. Atrial flutter with variable A–V block
    C. Sinus bradycardia with frequent PVCs
    D. Sinus tachycardia with frequent PACs

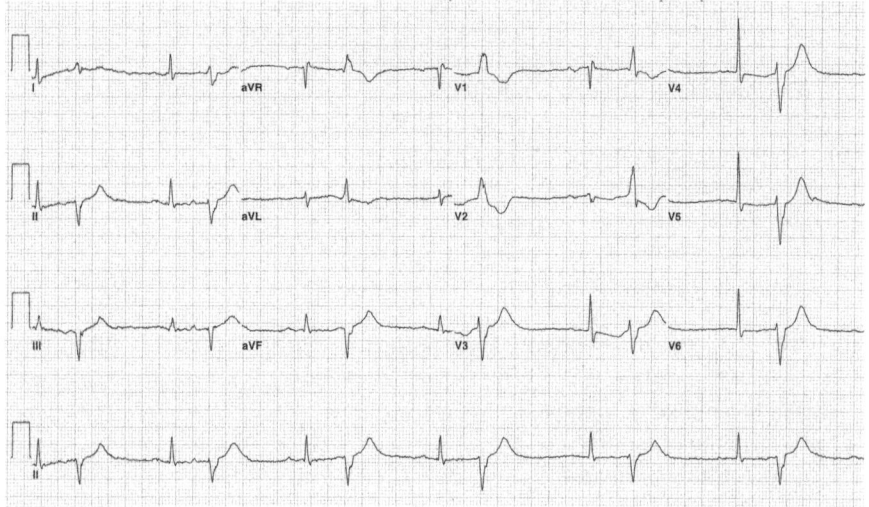

Fig. 4.6 Electrocardiogram

174. Inside the myocardial cell, ammonia is converted to an ammonium ion, which is trapped as:
    A. Fatty acid
    B. Glucose
    C. Glutamine
    D. Methionine

175. MRI and CT viability studies with intravenous contrast agents are based on evaluation of:
    A. Cell membrane integrity
    B. Contractile reserve
    C. Myocardial perfusion
    D. Scar tissue

176. Radiation exposure to patients from cardiac positron emission tomography (PET) perfusion imaging is approximately:
    A. 4–6 mSV
    B. 8–10 mSV
    C. 18–20 mSV
    D. 25–30 mSV

177. Which of the following radiotracers provides an alternative to Tc-99m pyrophosphate imaging for the detection of acute infarction?
    A. Tc-99m sestamibi
    B. F-18 fluorodeoxyglucose
    C. Tc-99m glucarate
    D. Tl-201 thallous chloride

178. Cardiac amyloidosis involves the deposition into the myofibril's:
    A. Amino acids
    B. Fatty acids
    C. Glycogen
    D. Leucocytes

179. A major source of error in SPECT reconstruction is data filtering. Filters that are too coarse may result in increase of:
    A. False positive studies
    B. True positive studies
    C. False negative studies
    D. False positive studies

180. The rate of perceived patient exertion readings of 14–16 on a Borg scale approximate/describe:
    A. Anaerobic threshold
    B. A patient's maximum exercise capacity
    C. Very hard exercise level
    D. Fairly light level of exercise

181. Myocardial extraction efficiency of Tl-201:
    A. Decreases at very low rate and at very high flow rates
    B. Increases at very low rate and at very high flow rates
    C. Decreases at very low rates, increases at very high flow rates
    D. Increases at very low rates, decreases at very high flow rates

182. The SPECT myocardial perfusion radiotracers show a significant roll-off at coronary blood flow levels exceeding:
    A. 0.5 mL/min/g
    B. 1.5 mL/min/g
    C. 2.0 mL/min/g
    D. 2.5 mL/min/g

183. Moore's correction method, the 3-window transformation method, and the convolution correction method are used for the correction of:
    A. Attenuation
    B. Dual-isotope cross talk
    C. Motion artifacts
    D. Scatter

184. Which of the following statements describing properties of nitrogen-13 (N-13) ammonia as a tracer of myocardial blood flow is CORRECT?
    A. The first-pass radiotracer extraction of N-13 ammonia is low at resting flows
    B. High contrast myocardial perfusion images are obtained within 1–5 min after the N-13 ammonia administration
    C. N-13 ammonia activity concentrations linearly increase with changes in myocardial blood flow
    D. At flows of 2.5–3.0 mL/min/g, further flow increases are associated with progressively smaller increases in myocardial N-13 ammonia concentrations

185. Which of the following serves as a metabolic coupler between oxygen consumption and coronary blood flow?
    A. Adenosine
    B. Dipyridamole
    C. Dobutamine
    D. Regadenoson

186. Figure 4.7 presents a screenshot of a standard LAO view MUGA scan. The arrow is pointing to the:
    A. Left atrium
    B. Left ventricle
    C. Right atrium
    D. Right ventricle

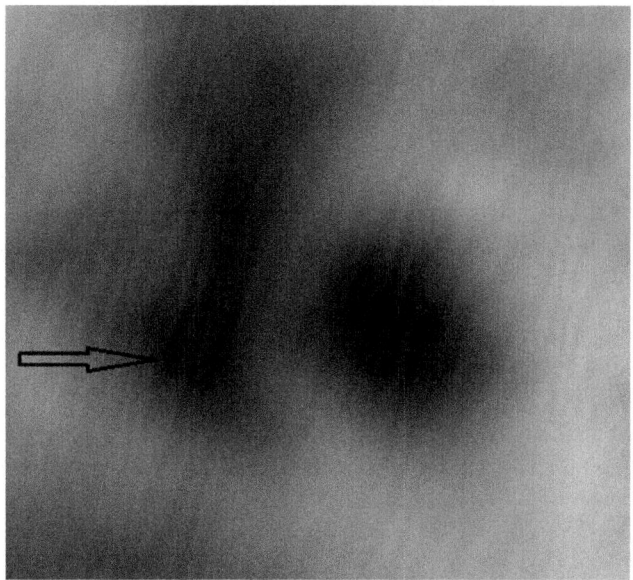

Fig. 4.7 MUGA scan

187. Cataract formation and skin damage due to radiation exposure are examples of:
    A. Deterministic effects
    B. Fatal effects
    C. Fetal effects
    D. Stochastic effects

188. Which of the following radiotracers has been used for the detection of necrosis associated with myocarditis and heart transplant rejection?
    A. I-131 MIBG
    B. In-111 labeled antimyosin antibody
    C. I-123 BMIPP
    D. F-18 fluorodeoxyglucose

189. Which of the following statements describing the radiation from a sealed radioactive source and an X-ray tube used in transmission computed tomography (TCT) is CORRECT:
    A. The radiation from a radioactive source is polyenergetic gamma-rays and polychromatic X-ray from an X-ray tube
    B. The radiation from a radioactive source is monoenergetic gamma-rays and polychromatic X-ray from an X-ray tube
    C. The radiation from a radioactive source is monoenergetic gamma-rays and monochromatic X-ray from an X-ray tube
    D. The radiation from a radioactive source is polyenergetic gamma-rays and monochromatic X-ray from an X-ray tube

190. The third stage of the Modified Bruce protocol corresponds to:
    A. The first stage of the Standard Bruce Test protocol
    B. The second stage of the Standard Bruce Test protocol
    C. The third stage of the Standard Bruce Test protocol
    D. The fourth stage of the Standard Bruce Test protocol

191. SPECT imaging data in patients with left ventricle hypertrophy (LVH) have a risk stratification value similar to that in patients:
    A. With left bundle branch block
    B. With hypertrophic cardiomyopathy
    C. With anterior wall attenuation
    D. Without left ventricle hypertrophy

192. According to the ASNC SPECT MPI guidelines peak pixel activity in the LV myocardium in an anterior planar projection for a Tc-99m should exceed:
    A. 10 cts
    B. 20 cts
    C. 100 cts
    D. 200 cts

193. Which of the following filters is described as the adaptive filter?
    A. Butterworth filter
    B. Hamming filter
    C. Parzen filter
    D. Wiener filter

194. Which of the following myocardial perfusion tracers is NOT accumulated in the myocardium?
    A. N-13 ammonia
    B. O-15 water
    C. Rb-82
    D. Tl-201

195. Pulmonary embolism, dissecting aneurysm, and pericardial tamponade can result in a cardiovascular complication described as:
    A. Anaphylactic shock
    B. Distributive shock
    C. Hypovolemic shock
    D. Obstructive shock

196. The rationale for prone imaging and reducing diaphragmatic attenuation is that:
    A. The heart shifts slightly superior and the diaphragm is more inferior in the prone position
    B. The heart shifts slightly inferior and the diaphragm is more superior in the prone position
    C. The heart and the diaphragm shifts slightly superior in the prone position
    D. The heart and the diaphragm are more inferior in the prone position

197. The principle stating that the exposure of individuals should be subject to dose restrictions designed to ensure that no individual is exposed to an unacceptable radiation risk is called:
    A. Contraindication
    B. Justification
    C. Limitation
    D. Optimization

198. All of the following statements correctly describe the morphology of the T wave EXCEPT:
    A. The T wave is influenced by body position
    B. The T wave is influenced by myocardial ischemia
    C. The T wave is influenced by hyperventilation
    D. The T wave is a marker of myocardial ischemia

199. Motion that occurs when the heart is close to the detector:
    A. Is more likely to introduce image artifacts
    B. Produces the same artifacts as if the camera was far away
    C. Is less likely to introduce image artifacts
    D. Doesn't produce image artifacts

200. The resolution recovery method includes the:
    A. Attenuation coefficients
    B. Center-of-rotation angulation
    C. Collimator-detector response
    D. Multihead registration algorithm

201. A 73-year-old male patient with a history of percutaneous coronary intervention (Fig. 4.8). Which of the following correctly describe cardiac CT findings?
    A. Calcium deposit
    B. Normal LAD
    C. Stent with restenosis
    D. Stent without restenosis

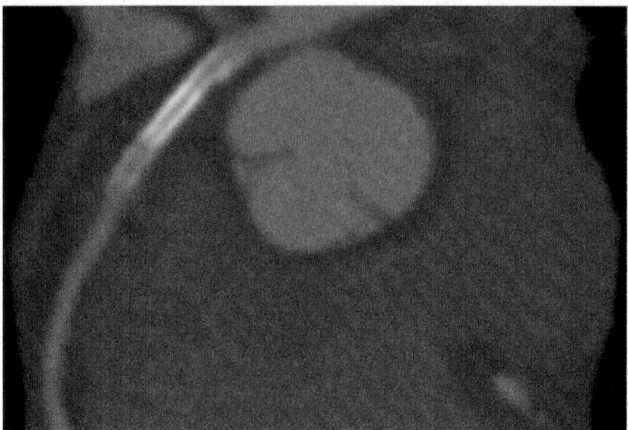

Fig. 4.8 Cardiac CT

202. Which of the following methods was developed purposely to solve the problem of EF estimation in small hearts?
    A. The cardiac function method (CAFU)
    B. The Gated SPECT Cardiac Quantification (GSCQ) method
    C. The Layer of Maximum Count (LMC) method
    D. The left ventricular global thickening fraction (LVGTF) method

203. Which of the following parameters describe the sum of infarcted or hibernating myocardium?
    A. Ejection Fraction (EF)
    B. Summed Stress Score (SSS)
    C. Summed Rest Score (SRS)
    D. Summed Difference Score (SDS)

204. Which of the following are used to improve the interpretation of polar maps derived from MPI studies?
    A. Dose-weighting and distance-weighting methods
    B. Volume-weighting and dose-weighting approaches
    C. Volume-weighting and distance-weighting methods
    D. Weight-weighting and height-weighting approaches

205. The RegEx trial- a randomized, double-blind, placebo- and active controlled pilot MPI study-combined:
    A. A selective A_{2A} agonist with high-level exercise
    B. Dipyridamole with low-level exercise
    C. A selective A_{2A} agonist with low-level exercise
    D. Adenosine with low-level exercise

206. In left dominance, the posterior descending artery PDA stems from the:
    A. Distal LCX
    B. Proximal LCX
    C. Mid RCA
    D. Distal RCA

207. A new prospectively gated axial (PGA) CT acquisition protocol has been introduced to reduce the radiation dose by utilizing only:
    A. The mid-systolic phase of the cardiac cycle
    B. The mid-diastolic phase of the cardiac cycle
    C. The end-systolic phase of the cardiac cycle
    D. The end-diastolic phase of the cardiac cycle

208. Which of the following is the best form of arterial access during cardiac cauterization?
    A. A percutaneous brachial artery
    B. A percutaneous carotid artery
    C. A percutaneous femoral artery
    D. A percutaneous radial artery

209. Which of the following is common and strong predictor of clinically significant coronary heart disease and established markers of an adverse cardiovascular prognosis as determined by stress MPI?
    A. Asthma bronchiale
    B. Erectile dysfunction
    C. Gastric ulcer
    D. Thrombophlebitis

210. A 55-year-old man with recurrent episodes of exertional chest pain/dyspnea and family history of CAD. He had hypertension, diabetes, and hypercholesterolemia for 5 years; his coronary angiogram (Fig. 4.9) showed lesion on the proximal:
    A. LCx-50 % stenosis
    B. LCx-100 % stenosis
    C. LAD-50 % stenosis
    D. LAD-100 % stenosis

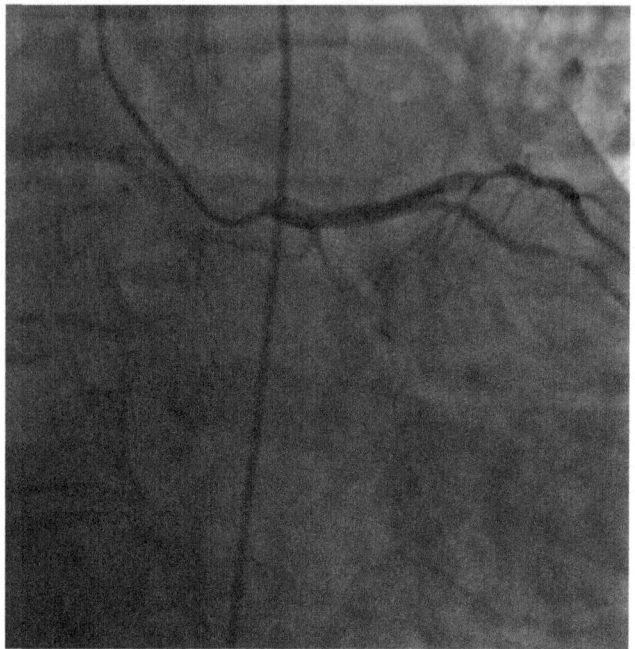

Fig. 4.9 Coronary angiogram

211. The blood pressure on the right side of circulation is approximately:
    A. Equal to that on the left
    B. 20 % of that on the left
    C. 50 % of that on the left
    D. 80 % of that on the left

212. Genetic cells divide during the process of:
    A. Apoptosis
    B. Meiosis
    C. Mitosis
    D. Symbiosis

213. Which of the following statements correctly describes the prognostic value of SPECT-MPI findings in patients with coronary artery disease?
    A. Perfusion defect size is most predictive of future myocardial infarction
    B. Perfusion defect reversibility is the strongest predictor of mortality
    C. LV ejection fraction is the strongest predictor of mortality
    D. LV ejection fraction is most predictive of future myocardial infarction

214. Boundary detection algorithms to define the endocardial and epicardial borders for LV volume calculations are adversely affected by all of the following EXCEPT:
    A. High background activity
    B. Low tracer dose administration
    C. Prior infarction
    D. Tracer selection

215. Which of the following arrhythmias is the most common in congenital heart disease patients?
    A. Atrial flutter
    B. Atrial tachycardia
    C. Ventricular bradycardia
    D. Ventricular tachycardia

Answers

1. C. Post-stress ejection fraction >35 %

   Post-stress ejection fraction <35 % and a stress-induced moderate perfusion defects with left ventricular dilatation, or increased lung uptake, also identifies patients with high risk annual mortality.
   (Gibbons 2000)

2. A. Apical thinning

   Phantom studies demonstrate that apical thinning is not simply an anatomical feature but can also be an artifact introduced by the use of attenuation correction.
   (Wheat and Currie 2006)

3. C. Myocardial ischemic memory imaging

   Abnormalities in fatty acid metabolism, following an ischemic episode, may persist long after perfusion has returned to normal imaging of fatty acid metabolism that may allow detection and evaluation of recent ischemia (ischemic memory).
   (Bonow et al. 2011)

4. A. Markedly impacts the attenuation correction when compared with a transmission scan

   A fast helical CT scan is acquired during a fraction of the respiratory cycle while the PET image is acquired over the whole respiratory cycle; a potential misalignment between emission and transmission data creates the risk of incomplete correction and consequently artificial perfusion defects.
   (Martinez-Möller et al. 2007)

5. C. Increased wall tension

   Increased subendocardial wall tension causes a relative increase in myocardial oxygen demand in the subendocardium.
   (Bonow et al. 2011)

6. D. Gating doesn't help to differentiate ischemic from nonischemic, dilated cardiomyopathy

   Even though both the perfusion and the LV function are abnormal in patients with ischemic cardiomyopathy, LV dysfunction is present without any significant perfusion abnormalities in patients with nonischemic cardiomyopathy.
   (Paul and Nabi 2004)

7. D. About 6–8 min

The pharmacological effects of dipyridamole persist for 15–30 min; however, it may last as long as 60 min. Dipyridamole is an indirect coronary vasodilator that works by increasing intravascular adenosine levels—the increase in coronary blood flow induced by dipyridamole is less predictable than that of adenosine.
(Iskandrian et al. 2003)

8. A. Bayes' theorem

For a given positive test result, the posttest probability of disease may be distinctly lower in a patient with a very low pretest probability of disease. However, in a patient with positive test result and with a much higher pretest probability of disease, the posttest probability of disease would be distinctly higher.
(Bayes theorem Accessed May 17, 2012)

9. C. False negative studies

This potential problem due to over smoothing may be particularly challenging in detecting small or non-transmural defects clinically.
(Cherry et al. 2003)

10. D. Increased muscle oxygen extraction

Before the start of exercise, in healthy persons, the net effect is increased resting cardiac output.
(Bonow et al. 2011)

11. B. Tc-99m teboroxime

Its most remarkable feature is the high myocardial extraction fraction, which is well correlated with the coronary blood flow. The tracer has been approved by the FDA as a myocardial perfusion imaging agent but the extremely rapid myocardial washout limits its use in every day clinical practice.
(Bonow et al. 2011)

12. B. Fourier space

Fourier space is the space in which the Fourier transform of a function is expressed. Fourier theory states that visual images can be expressed as a sum of a series of sinusoids. In the case of imaging, these are sinusoidal variations that are appreciated as the brightness across the image.
(Zubal and Wisniewski 1997)

13. B. structural variations of the myocardium—the muscular septum is merging with the membranous septum

Normal "dropout" of the basal septum can be seen in the most basal short-axis tomograms and the basal septal portion in the horizontal long-axis view.
(Bonow et al. 2011)

14. C. Drift of the contents of abdominal cavity

Wander of the thoracic contents follows response to changes in lung volume as a result of the administration of a pharmacologic stressing agent.
(Ho and Reddy 2011)

15. B. Improvement in function

Besides improvement in the LVEF, improvement in symptoms and exercise capacity may be clinically relevant. The obtainable evidence suggests that 20–30% of the left ventricle needs to be viable to allow improvement in the LVEF.
(Schinkel et al. 2007)

16. D. Anaerobic threshold

The term "anaerobic" means "without air" or "without oxygen." Anaerobic metabolism occurs at high intensity exercise and a high rate of work for a short period of time, e.g., sprinting, heavy weight lifting.
(Bonow et al. 2011)

17. C. 7 years postirradiation

The timing of the appearance of radiation-induced cancers varies, with a mean incidence for thyroid and bone cancers occurring at about 5 years postirradiation and 20 or more years for most other cancers.
(ICRP 2001 Accessed July 1, 2012)

18. D. None of the above

The USPSTF concludes that the current evidence is insufficient to assess the balance of risks and benefits of screening with resting or exercise ECG for the prediction of CHD events in asymptomatic adults at intermediate or high risk for CHD events.
(Moyer 2012)

19. B. A high-grade coronary stenosis

The degree of the poststress regional or global dysfunction correlates with the severity of the ischemia; stress-induced stunning is more sensitive than a resting and stress wall motion abnormality and is highly specific for a severe angiographic stenosis.
(Emmett et al. 2002)

20. C. Perceived patient exertion

The Borg scale is based on the physical sensations a person experiences during physical activity, including increased heart rate, increased respiration or breathing rate, increased sweating, and muscle fatigue. The scale is linear, with values of 9 for very light, 11 for fairly light, 13 for somewhat hard, 15 for hard, 17 for very hard, and 19 for very, very hard perceived exertion.
(CDC Accessed September 20, 2012)

21. D. The maximal 85 % of age-predicted heart rate is reached

The age-predicted HRmax equation (i.e., 220—age) is generally employed as a foundation for prescribing exercise programs, as a measure for achieving maximal exertion, and as a clinical guide during diagnostic exercise testing.
(Burrell and MacDonald 2006)

22. C. Inverse Fourier transform

Inverse Fourier transform transfers the frequency group back into the x, y coordinate system, reconstructing the image.
(Zubal and Wisniewski 1997)

23. A. Scaling method

This method works fine for tissue whose attenuation is primarily Compton scatter; however, it is not effective in tissue of high atomic number, where the photoelectric absorption is a greater component of attenuation.
(Fleming 1989)

24. B. Is less than the attenuation of the 80- to 140-keV photons emitted by SPECT radiotracers

The TOTAL attenuation may in fact be greater for PET—two coincident photons need to travel across the whole body to reach their respective detectors—than for SPECT.
(Bonow et al. 2011)

25. B. Intracoronary steal

Intracoronary steal (from endocardium to subepicardial territory) occurs because of higher vasodilator reserve in the subepicardial vessels compared to subendocardial vessels.
(Akinboboye et al. 2001)

26. D. A simulated attenuation correction

Regardless of technical challenges, the application of attenuation correction has been shown to add to the diagnostic accuracy of stress myocardial perfusion SPECT studies, primarily by improving specificity.
(Bonow et al. 2011)

27. B. Ventricular pacemaker

Atrial and ventricular pacing can be seen on the electrocardiogram (ECG) as a pacing stimulus (spike) followed by a P wave or QRS complex, respectively. The ECG has the ability to show normal and abnormal pacemaker function. An implantable cardioverter-defibrillator (ICD) device can sense potentially lethal ventricular arrhythmias and deliver appropriate electrical therapy, including defibrillatory shocks.
(Goldberger 2006)

28. C. Atherosclerosis

Whether these promising results in animals can be transformed to the clinical setting of patients with potentially unstable atherosclerosis is the subject of a current study. SPECT has been used to image apoptosis, by targeting annexin A5 in rabbits, and to track monocytes in experimental mouse atherosclerosis.
(Jaffer and Narula 2009)

29. D. 9 mSv in 50 % of patients

Among others, ASNC recommends that the clinical indications and physical stature of each patient should be reviewed, and the best combination of radio-tracers and protocols used:
Radionuclides with shorter half-life perform stress-only testing and use weight-based dosing.
(Cerqueira et al. 2010)

30. C. Increase perfusion

Oxygen extraction in the coronary circulation is already nearly maximal at rest. The heart is an aerobic organ with modest capacity to produce energy through anaerobic metabolism.
(Bonow et al. 2011)

31. B. In favor of applying attenuation correction in addition to ECG gating with SPECT MPI

This recommendation, however, presumes that personnel are highly knowledgeable about the technique and its stringent quality control when applying the attenuation correction methodology.
(Hendel et al. 2002)

32. B. Fractionation

D. Prolongation
According to the ASNC imaging guidelines, the study should not be attempted if those sites are not accessible.
(ASNC Accessed June 17, 2012)

33. B. Attenuation correction

Artifacts due to soft tissue attenuation may be improved by various techniques of attenuation correction. Attenuation correction methods include either line source or computed tomographic (CT) techniques.
(Zaidi and Hasegawa 2003)

34. C. CT scanner "freezes" the heart, lungs, and liver at one point in the respiratory cycle, whereas the PET emission data are averaged over many respiratory cycles. One problem of using fast CT scans for attenuation correction is the motion of the organs during respiration—methods using respiratory gating are under investigation.

(Bonow et al. 2011)

35. C. Indicates the presence of L–R shunt

This shunted activity begins to arrive during the downslope of the primary curve, resulting in a blunting of the rate of descent of the curve.
(MacDonald and Burrell 2008)

36. D. Warm-up phenomenon

Change for the better on the second test is linked to the degree of myocardial ischemia produced on the first test, and commonly, myocardial ischemia of more than moderate intensity is needed to produce the warm-up response.
(Bogaty et al. 2003)

37. C. cm^{-1}

Units of cycles per centimeter, or cm^{-1}, describe the number of waves (frequencies) that fit per centimeter across the image; units of cycles per pixel or $pixel^{-1}$ can also be used to describe the cut-off. Conversions can be easily made from per centimeter to per pixel, by correctly multiplying or dividing by the image pixel size.
(Zubal and Wisniewski 1997)

38. A. Arterial-venous oxygen difference

$MVO_2 = CBF \times (CaO_2 - CvO_2)$
where CBF = coronary blood flow (ml/min), and $(CaO_2 - CvO_2)$ is the arterial-venous oxygen content difference (ml O_2/ml blood).
(Klabunde Accessed July 21, 2012)

39. C. 10 days

The effective half-life, based on both the radiological decay and biological clearance of thallium-201 in the body, is about 2.3 days.
(Thrall and Taveras 2006)

40. C. A moderate level of intensity

The Borg scale of perceived patient exertion is based on the physical sensations a person experiences during physical activity, including increased heart rate, increased respiration or breathing rate, increased sweating, and muscle fatigue.
(Bonow et al. 2011)

41. C. Motion that occurs when the heart is close to the detector is less likely to create image artifacts

Examination of the projection data in a cine loop format is generally the best way to become aware of cardiac motion.
(Ibrahim and DiFilippo 2006)

42. A. Atrioventricular conduction delay

Activation of A1 receptors can induce transient heart block in the atrioventricular (AV) node (cell hyperpolarization by increasing outward K+ flux); for this reason adenosine is used in the management of supraventricular arrhythmia.
(Heller et al. Accessed July 22, 2011)

43. D. Horizontal long-axis view

The horizontal long axis is displayed with serial tomograms beginning at the inferior surface of the heart and progressing toward the superior surface: the cardiac apex at the top and the cardiac base at the bottom, with the left ventricle to the viewer's right and the right ventricle to the viewer's left.
(SNM.AHA.ACR. 1992)

44. B.Rb-82 chloride

Rubidium chloride, Rb-82, injection must be administered only with an appropriate infusion system capable of meeting the recommended performance characteristics.
(Rubidium Rb-82 Generator Accessed July 13, 2012)

45. C. Myocardial perfusion

The microbubbles stay in the vascular space and perform like red cells in terms of flow and can be used to visualize myocardial perfusion directly.
(Schinkel et al. 2007)

46. B. Anteriorly or laterally

Just as supine position may produce an inferior and or inferior-lateral wall defect, prone imaging may result in septal and or anterior-septal wall defect—likely due to the fact that the septum lies closer to the detector in the prone position.
(Hayes et al. 2003)

47. D. The half-life of terminal phase is approximately 2 h

    An initial phase parallels with the onset of the pharmacodynamic response
    and an intermediate phase corresponds to loss of the pharmacodynamic effect.
    (Astellas Accessed July 28, 2012)

48. D. Oxygen

    The oxygen requirement of the myocardium, as assessed by the rate of oxygen
    consumed (MVO_2), is determined by the heart rate, left ventricle contractility,
    and left ventricular volume.
    (Weber and Janicki 1979)

49. C. An electronic signal

    A semiconductor CZT mixes the functions of scintillation crystals and PM
    tubes, producing smaller, more proficient devices with high count rates and
    high-energy resolution.
    (Travin 2011)

50. A. ≤ -11

    DTS was developed to provide accurate diagnostic and prognostic informa-
    tion for the evaluation of patients with suspected coronary heart disease.
    (Mark et al. 1987)

51. B. 10–15 min after injection

    The rate of thallium clearance from myocardium is related to the concentra-
    tion gradient between myocytes and the blood levels of thallium.
    (Baggish and Boucher 2008)

52. C. Tc-99m diethylamine triamine pentaacetic acid

    Tc-99m pertechnetate and other technetium-based compounds, such as the
    technetium perfusion agents: sestamibi and tetrofosmin are also appropriate.
    (ASNC Accessed June 17, 2012)

53. C. Advanced image reconstruction techniques

    Several "resolution recovery" processing software techniques have been
    developed to incorporate a sophisticated resolution recovery method into iter-
    ative reconstruction, accounting for collimator geometry, distance to the
    patient, as well as adding noise suppression.
    (Travin 2011)

54. A. Balanced ischemia

    Patients with multivessel CAD may display uniform reduction in flow reserve,
    and the relative perfusion data from SPECT may fail to recognize this "bal-
    anced" ischemia.
    (Bonow et al. 2011)

55. B. Contractile reserve

Nuclear imaging by SPECT is based on evaluating perfusion, cell membrane integrity, and intactness of mitochondria with Tl-201- or Tc-99m-labeled agents.
(Schinkel et al. 2007)

56. B. The flux of X-ray photons from a conventional sealed source is much higher than typical X-ray tube

The primary differences between a sealed radioactive source (e.g., Gd-153) and an X-ray tube include the type of radiation used and the photon emission rate that dictates the quality-control (QC) protocols that are required.
(Holly et al. 2010)

57. B. 10 h

The decision to discontinue nursing after administration of Lexiscan, or not to administer Lexiscan, should take into account the importance of the drug to the mother. Based on the pharmacokinetics of Lexiscan, it should be cleared 10 h after administration.
(Astellas Accessed July 28, 2012)

58. B. Disease progression bias

To eliminate "disease progression bias" in a SPECT /angio correlation study, only studies where the SPECT and catheter angiography exams were done within 30 days of each other should be included.
(Iskandar 2012)

59. A. 0.7 % per year

In patients with a normal study, the rate of cardiac death or nonfatal MI occurring during an average follow-up of 2 years is 0.7 % per year—this data applies across a broad spectrum of isotopes, protocols, and stressors.
(Ficaro and Hansen Accessed April 13, 2010)

60. C. Heart rate recovery

Abnormal heart rate recovery reflects decreased vagal tone and is associated with increased mortality. HRR can be calculated from the formula: HRR=HRpeak-HR 1 min later. When the postexercise phase includes an upright cool-down, a value of 12 beats/min or less is abnormal.
(Bonow et al. 2011)

61. D. The camera sensitivity

Transmission source decay, higher injected activities, and larger body sizes all tend to decrease the transmission-to-cross-talk value (TCR).
(Holly et al. 2010)

62. C. A2b

Adenosine A1 receptors are present in the sinus node and atrioventricular (AV) node and mediate diminished heart rate and AV nodal conduction.
(Dilsizian et al. 2009)

63. D. Stress radionuclide MPI

Since the ECG is interpretable, appropriate use criteria recommend stress radionuclide myocardial perfusion imaging over exercise ECG.
(Hendel et al. 2009)

64. B. Mitochondria

New PET perfusion imaging tracers bind to the mitochondrial complex I of the electron transport chain with high affinity. They demonstrate good uptake in the heart due to its high density of mitochondria.
(Ghosh et al. 2010)

65. C. Triphasic response

Biphasic response is identified when initial improvement is followed by worsening of wall motion; No change pattern is recognized when there is no change in wall motion during the entire study.
(Schinkel et al. 2007)

66. D. Normal supine-only studies

The prognostic value of prone imaging was assessed in a series of 3,834 patients; patients with an inferior defect also had prone imaging. At a mean follow-up of 24 months, patients with normal prone imaging had a low risk of subsequent cardiac events that was comparable to the risk in patients with normal supine-only studies.
(Hayes et al. 2003)

67. C. Renal afferent arterioles

Adenosine is a powerful vasodilator in most vascular beds, except in renal afferent arterioles and hepatic veins, where it produces vasoconstriction.
(Astellas Accessed March 28, 2012)

68. D. $\geq 80\%$

In critical stenosis, regardless of the myocardial blood flow (MBF) level under resting conditions, any increase of cardiac workload and oxygen demand that cannot be met by an adequate increase in MBF, consequently, leads to demand ischaemia. Patients with LV dysfunction and CFR <1.49 on 13NH3 MBF quantification had a worse survival rate.
(Ghosh et al. 2010)

69. B. Mitochondria

In addition to supplying cellular energy, mitochondria are implicated in other tasks such as signaling, cellular differentiation, cell death, as well as the control of the cell cycle and cell growth.
(Voet et al. 2006)

70. B. Premature atrial contractions

Presence of LV hypertrophy, digitalis therapy, and ST depression at rest also complicate interpretation of ECG changes and preclude use of exercise ECG for noninvasive stress testing.
(Iskandrian and Garcia 2012)

71. C. CsI(Tl) crystals

Cadmium zinc telluride or CsI(Tl) crystals deliver significantly more information for each detected gamma ray.
(Erlandsson et al. 2009)

72. B. The percentage R–L shunt

The existence of an R–L shunt results in greater activity surfacing within the systemic organs. Normally only about 3 % of the activity is seen outside the lungs.
(MacDonald and Burrell 2008)

73. B. Atrial flutter with variable A-V block

Atrial flutter has a single, stable reentrant pathway, and as a result all flutter (F) waves look exactly the same in both shape and duration. Atrial wave cycle length—F–F intervals— is ≥ 180 ms. These rapid contractions are slowed when they reach the AV node—often only every second or third contraction ever reaches the ventricle.
(Goldberger 2006)

74. C. GLUT1 and GLUT 4

The tracer is transported into the myocyte by the same sarcolemmal glucose transporters, (GLUT1 and GLUT4), as glucose and is phosphorylated to F-18 FDG-6-phosphate by hexokinase.
(Ghosh et al. 2010)

75. B. Endothelial function

Preserved endothelial function permits appropriate flow-mediated vasodilation during stress, and consequently reduces the impact of an angiographically demonstrated stenosis on the downstream myocardial perfusion.
(Bonow et al. 2011)

76. D. Stunning

    The incidence and duration of postischemic dysfunction correlates with the number of diseased coronary vessels—poststress dysfunction resolves quickly when most patients with single-vessel CAD stopped exercising.
    (Toba et al. 2004)

77. B. Low frequencies

    This filter enhances high frequencies by multiplying all frequencies by a value proportional to the frequency.
    (English and Brown 1990)

78. C. MRI

    GSPECT tends to overestimate EDV and ESV compared with MRI at higher volumes and underestimate LVEF when LVEF is very low.
    (Constantine et al. 2004)

79. C. RNA-derived EF is based on geometric assumptions

    RNA-derived EF is based on count changes.
    (Iskandrian and Garcia 2012)

80. C. Sixfold

    The pulmonary vascular bed can hold as much as a sixfold increase in cardiac output, with only modest increases in pulmonary pressure. Pulmonary blood flow is not a restraining factor of peak exercise capacity in healthy patients.
    (Akinpelu Accessed October 11, 2012)

81. B. Nyquist

    The Nyquist frequency, also called the Nyquist limit, is the highest frequency that can be coded at a given sampling rate, in order to be able to fully reconstruct the signal.
    (Christian et al. 2004)

82. B. A reduction of 8–10 mm Hg in systolic and diastolic blood pressure and reflex increase in heart rate by 10 and 20 beats/min

    A blunted heart rate response may be observed in patients who are taking beta blockers or in diabetic patients with underlying autonomic insufficiency.
    (Dilsizian et al. 2009)

83. B. Systolic wall thickening

    The count density is linearly related to the expansion in wall thickness (brightness) during myocardial contraction.
    (Paul and Nabi 2004)

84. C. An electrocardiograph

    The cardiac series is examined with an ECG; the phase is divided into a pre-determined, commonly eight number of bins between sequential R–R waves. (Ho and Reddy 2011)

85. C. At moderate risk for CAD

    The American College of Cardiology guidelines for determining the pretest likelihood of CAD in patients with chest pain were established according to their sex, age, and type of chest discomfort.
    (Gibbons et al. 1999)

86. D. After the injection of the radioisotope, the milk can be collected and given to the infant

    There is no need to throw away the milk. The physician or RSO should determine how long the milk should be kept for adequate decay.
    (Wackers et al. 2004)

87. C. Adenosine triphosphate (ATP)

    ATP is the primary energy source in cells for their transport systems and many enzymes. Most ATP is hydrolyzed to ADP, which can be further dephosphory-lated to AMP.
    (Zaret and Beller 2005)

88. B. Steal

    As a result of coronary steal, flow to the bed supplied by a severe epicardial stenosis, may decrease compared with resting flow. The diminished supply may create supply-demand mismatch and true myocardial ischemia, with ECG ST segment depression.
    (Dilsizian et al. 2009)

89. B. Heart-to-mediastinum ratio

    An abnormal heart-to-mediastinum ratio (H/M) is an independent and more potent predictor than LVEF for sudden cardiac death in heart failure patients.
    (Zaret and Beller 2005)

90. C. Maximum exercise capacity

    Maximum exercise capacity can be evaluated using markers such as maximal exercise duration, maximal MET level achieved, maximum workload achieved, or maximum heart rate and heart rate–blood pressure product.
    (Akinpelu Accessed October 11, 2012)

91. B. 40 % of myocardial perfusion studies in women

Breast size, breast tissue density, and breast position relative to the heart may influence the amount and severity of soft tissue attenuation.
(Manglos et al. 1993)

92. D. Superior vena cava

The injection should occur at a site with minimal distance to the right side of the heart; the right external jugular vein is best fitted to help maintain the bolus, but for practical purposes, an antecubital vein is often substituted.
(MacDonald and Burrell 2008)

93. B. Poststress LVEF is the best predictor of cardiac death, whereas the amount of ischemia is the best predictor of nonfatal infarction

Patients with an LVEF $\geq$45 %, or an ESV $\leq$70 mL, had a lower mortality rate, despite severe perfusion abnormalities, whereas patients with an LVEF <45 %, or an ESV >70 mL, had a higher mortality rate, even with mild-to-moderate perfusion abnormalities.
(Sharir et al. 1999)

94. B. A guess of the image

On the basis of supposing that the activity is at the locations in the guessed image, scanning is imitated to produce a simulated data set.
(Ho and Reddy 2011)

95. A. Bayes' theorem

The pretest probability of disease is evaluated on the basis of patient history, physical examination, and risk factor assessment.
(Koller 2002)

96. A. diastolic blood pressure > 90 mm Hg

In case of severe chest pain associated with ST depression of 2 mm or greater, signs of poor perfusion, or there are technical problems with the monitoring, the test should be terminated.
(ASNC Accessed April 07, 2012)

97. B. phase analysis

Diastolic dyssynchrony is considerably more widespread than systolic dyssynchrony and is linked to cardiac risk factors and diastolic dysfunction in patients with end-stage renal disease (ESRD) and normal LVEF.
(Iskandrian and Garcia 2012)

98. D. A reduction of presynaptic norepinephrine uptake and increase in postsynaptic β-adrenoceptor density

    I-123 MIBG imaging has demonstrated drug-induced changes in cardiac adrenergic activity.
    (Caldwell et al. 2008)

99. D. Increase in the LVEF, a decrease in the ESV

    Post-CABG patients generally show abnormal wall motion of the septum, despite no significant myocardial damage.
    (Paul and Nabi 2004)

100. D. A patient's maximum exercise capacity

    18–20 ratings on the Borg scale is an extremely strenuous exercise level. For most people this is the most strenuous exercise they have ever experienced.
    (Bonow et al. 2011)

101. A. Angina like chest pain, B. Fall in blood pressure, D. Substantial ST depression at low work rate

    Interpretation of exercise stress tests should always include exercise capacity, and clinical, hemodynamic, and ECG response.
    (Banerjee et al. 2012)

102. B. Pulmonary background is reduced in the upright position

    The selection of upright versus supine positioning depends on the clinical situation. Pulmonary background is diminished in the upright position, which improves study quality.
    (ASNC Accessed June 17, 2012)

103. D. Proximal location of stenosis

    History of myocardial infarction, extensive CAD, high-grade coronary stenosis, and presence of regional wall motion abnormalities increase sensitivity of MPI.
    (Beller and Zaret 2000)

104. A. Change charge state

    Injected Rubidium flows through the coronary arteries into cardiac capillaries, where it can cross the capillary membrane into the cardiac tissue, alter its charge, and become trapped.
    (Ho and Reddy 2011)

105. B. Digoxin

    Resting ECG abnormalities may compromise the accuracy of diagnostic data from the ECG—down-slope ST segment depression; T wave inversion may be confused with myocardial ischemia.
    (Banerjee et al. 2012)

106. C. The CT source decays slower than a radionuclide source

The CT acquisition has a high flux, and for this reason the CT images will not be affected by cross-talk from the SPECT radionuclide. The CT source does not decay.
(O'Connor and Kemp 2006)

107. B. 66 %

End-diastolic volume (EDV), the volume of blood in each ventricle at the end of diastole, is usually about 120–130 mL, but can reach 200–250 mL in the normal heart.
(Zaret and Beller 2005)

108. D. 10 years

This tool is designed for adults aged 20 and older, who do not have heart disease or diabetes. The first Framingham Risk Score includes age, gender, LDL cholesterol, HDL cholesterol, blood pressure (and also whether the patient is treated or not for his/her hypertension), diabetes, and smoking.
(Third Report of the NCEP 2002)

109. C. An attenuation map

With an external source of radiation (e.g., technetium, gadolinium, or X-ray) positioned on one side of the patient and a detector on the other side and with known distance between the source and detector, the measured intensity data can calculated. By acquiring a number of these measures at different angles, a "map" of attenuation across the site of interest (thorax) is generated.
(Zaidi and Hasegawa 2003)

110. D. Ventilation gas analysis

CPET involves measurements of gas exchange, which primarily include oxygen uptake (i.e., VO_2), carbon dioxide output (VCO_2), minute ventilation, and anaerobic (lactic acid) threshold. Abnormal ventilatory and chronotropic responses to exercise are also predictors of outcome in patients with heart failure.
(Akinpelu Accessed October 11, 2012)

111. C. 30–45 min

Since dipyridamole has the longer half-life when compared to adenosine, patients can get a dipyridamole infusion and then undergo any level of supplemental exercise.
(Ahlberg et al. 2008)

112. B. Tc-99m sodium pertechnetate

Nuclear medicine assessment of an R–L shunt with a first pass analysis technique is based on demonstrating an early return of activity to the lungs after the initial flow there. If a L–R shunt is present, there will be recirculation of radiolabeled blood through the right heart, and onward to the lungs shortly after the initial bolus passes through the lungs, and long before the return of blood from the body.
(MacDonald and Burrell 2008)

113. D. Stress echocardiography is more accurate than stress MPI in patients with high body mass index

The diagnostic accuracy and prognostic value of the two methods are comparable; however, their relative accuracy may be influenced by certain patient characteristics.
(Papaioannou and Heller Accessed July 22, 2011)

114. B. Carbohydrate and fatty acid metabolism

The heart can use a variety of substrates including fatty acids, ketones, glucose, pyruvate, lactate, and amino acids to regenerate ATP depending upon availability.
(Zaret and Beller 2005)

115. B. Echocardiography

By assessing the motion of the heart wall, echocardiography can help detect the presence and assess the severity of coronary artery disease. Echocardiography is particularly indicated in patients with abnormal resting ECGs.
(Banerjee et al. 2012)

116. C. 250 mm Hg

The current ACC/AHA guidelines for exercise stress test (EST) describe a hypertensive response to exercise as one in which the systolic blood pressure rises to more than 250 mm Hg, or the diastolic blood pressure rises to more than 115 mm Hg.
(ACC/AHA 2002 Accessed September 21, 2012)

117. A. The A1-receptor agonism

Vascular smooth muscle relaxation, which leads to vasodilation, is a result of the A2-receptor agonism.
(Astellas Accessed March 28, 2012)

118. B. Ischemic equivalent

Examples of such findings include, but are not exclusive to, chest pain, chest tightness, burning, shoulder pain, palpitations, jaw pain, and new ECG abnormalities suggestive of ischemic heart disease.
(Appropriate Use Criteria (AUC) Accessed June 12, 2012)

119. C. Inversely related

Small structures in an image are said to have high frequency, and large objects are described as low frequency. The resolution ability of a camera is frequently described as the Nyquist frequency, that is, the highest frequency that the system can "see."
(Germano 2001)

120. C. Shortness of breath

According to the current ACC/AHA guidelines, shortness of breath, wheezing, leg cramps, or claudication and increasing nonanginal chest pain are relative indications to terminate an exercise stress test.
(Gibbons et al. 2002)

121. D. Selective A2A receptor agonists

Binodenoson and apadenoson, currently investigational, have been evaluated in phase 3 studies, are selective A2A adenosine receptor agonists that produces a similar degree of hyperemia to adenosine.
(Heller et al. Accessed July 22, 2011)

122. B. Myocardial viability

RNA can also provide information on LV/RV size, diastolic function, pulmonary blood volume, and can be used to assess dyssynchrony (nonsynchronized cardiac contractions).
(Zaret and Beller 2005)

123. C. Interventricular dyssynchrony

Dyssynchronous LV contraction (intraventricular dyssynchrony) leads to decreased ejection volume because blood relocates around the left ventricle from early activated segments to late activated segments.
(Yu et al. 2003)

124. A. 10 %

The uptake of FDG is flow independent, and the extraction across the capillary membranes in the course of a single pass is relatively small.
(Ho and Reddy 2011)

125. C. Ribosomes

Ribosomes link amino acids together in the order specified by messenger RNA (mRNA) molecules.
(Biology on Line Accessed July 23, 2012)

126. C. order

For lower-order filters, the transition between preserving frequencies and eliminating frequencies goes through a slower transition.
(Germano and Berman 2006)

127. D. Norepinephrine

Norepinephrine- a hormone and neurotransmitter-is secreted by the adrenal medulla and the nerve endings of the sympathetic nervous system to cause vasoconstriction and increases in HR, BP, and the glucose level of the blood.
(Bonow et al. 2011)

128. C. Nonfatal MI

"Hard events" definition also includes cardiac death or all-cause mortality. "Soft" cardiac events include revascularization and hospital admission for unstable angina or heart failure.
(Bonow et al. 2011)

129. A. Anginal symptoms

Exercise stress test in patients taking beta-blockers may have reduced diagnostic and prognostic value; however, according to the current ACC/AHA guidelines, discontinuing beta-blockers before EST is discouraged to avoid "rebound" hypertension or anginal symptoms.
(Gibbons et al. 2002)

130. C. 59–81 % and 61–73 % accordingly

Sensitivity and specificity varies depending on the study or article referenced. A meta-analysis of 58 consecutively published reports involving 11,691 patients showed a mean sensitivity of 67 % and a mean specificity of 72 %.
(Akinpelu Accessed October 11, 2012)

131. C. Glutamine synthase

Glutamine synthetase plays an essential role in the metabolism of nitrogen by catalyzing the condensation of glutamate and ammonia to form glutamine.
(Phelps 2004)

132. B. The atria from the ventricle

A caudal tilt may result in insertion of more left atrium than wanted, if the atrial-ventricular border is difficult to distinguish, as the superior aspect of the ROI may intrude into the left atrium.
(ASNC Accessed June 17, 2012)

133. B. 25 % of myocardial perfusion studies

Diaphragmatic attenuation is more common in men than in women. Localized diaphragmatic attenuation generally creates a fixed inferior defect (the position of the left hemidiaphragm is relatively stable and as a result, shifting attenuation artifacts are comparatively rare).
(Heller Accessed 18 June 2012)

134. B. F-18 fluoroethoxybenzovesamicol

Catecholamine analogues labeled with PET tracers such as F-18 fluorodopamine, C-11 epinephrine, C-11 metahydroxyephedrine, and C-11 phenylephrine are undergoing evaluation for their utility in assessing the cardiac sympathetic innervation.
(Takalkar et al. 2011)

135. C. Interventricular septum

The interventricular septum separates the left ventricle from the right ventricle. The left anterior oblique (LAO) acquisition is obtained at an angle that allows the best separation of the right and left ventricles (best septal or best separation view—approximately 45 0).
(Zaret and Beller 2005)

136. B. Right bundle branch block

Digoxin may also cause false positive ST depressions during exercise and is an indication for stress testing with imaging.
(Gibbons et al. 2002)

137. A. Fourier transform

The Fourier Transform is an important image processing tool which encodes all of the spatial frequencies present in an image into its sine and cosine components.
(Zubal and Wisniewski 1997)

138. D. Referral bias

The normalcy rate, used as a surrogate for specificity, is defined as the rate of normal perfusion scans in patients with 5 % likelihood of CAD on the basis of clinical and ECG stress test data.
(Ficaro and Hansen Accessed May, 22, 2012)

139. B. Excludes CAD as the cause of the cardiomyopathy

Extensive perfusion abnormalities in the setting of LV dysfunction are practically always associated with CAD rather than with DCM.
(Udelson et al. 2002)

140. B. 1.7 mph, 0 % grade

Low-level exercise is not recommended in patients with left bundle branch block (LBBB) or for patients with pacemakers.
(ASNC Accessed April 07, 2012)

141. B. A greater mitochondrial density

Mitochondria are the cellular energy generators. Enzymes within the mitochondria matrix are intended to oxidize the substrates within, in a cyclic manner.
(Fukumoto 2004)

142. C. Roll-off

The plateau effect limits the sensitivity of a tracer to detect CAD and reversible perfusion defects by reducing defect contrast; there is the potential to underestimate higher levels of coronary blood flow, and flow heterogeneity may not be observed.
(Husain 2007)

143. C. 5 % of breast uptake lesions are malignant

27 % of breast uptake lesions are malignant. Patients with ECFs, such as a hiatal hernia, pericardial effusion, pulmonary embolism, and gallbladder disease may have symptoms that can often simulate cardiac symptoms.
(Iskandrian and Garcia 2012)

144. D. Rubidium-82

Rubidium-82 is produced from a strontium-82 generator, and it is widely used in centers without on-site cyclotrons
(Takalkar et al. 2011)

145. C. Base (Fig. 4.10)

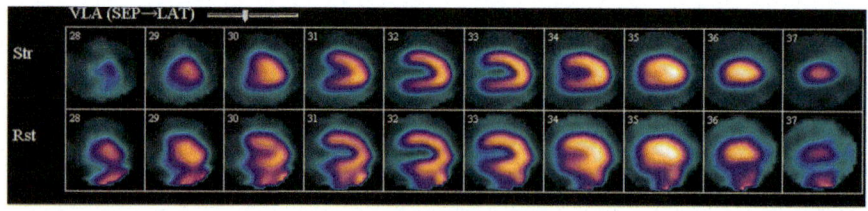

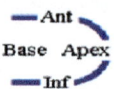

Fig. 4.10 SPECT MUGA

146. A. ECG-gated imaging

C. Prone imaging

F. Review of planar images

Several methods have been developed to improve artifact recognition, including breast markers (primarily used with planar imaging), prolonged acquisition time, and higher energy radiopharmaceuticals (technetium 99m versus thallium-201).

(Zaret and Beller 2005)

147. A. Brightness in the image

SPECT imaging of normal subjects should then generate a homogeneous brightness in black and white images, or color in color images in the myocardial pixels.

(Iskandrian and Garcia 2012)

148. C. Number of reversible perfusion defects increases

The extent of perfusion abnormalities detected by stress MPI has an important relationship with the subsequent likelihood of an adverse natural history outcome (cardiac death or nonfatal MI).

(Bonow et al. 2011)

149. B. Decreased lung Tl-201 uptake on Tl-201 scintigraphy

A large defect size (>20 % of the left ventricle), and defects in >1 coronary vascular supply regions suggestive of multivessel CAD and increased lung Tl-201 uptake, are indicators of future cardiac events.

(Beller and Zaret 2000)

150. D. Patients with three-vessel disease who have an abnormal exercise EF are less likely to benefit from revascularization

Patients who demonstrate a more normal EF response to exercise have a more positive natural history, and as a result, are less likely to benefit from revascularization.

(Ficaro and Hansen Accessed June 01, 2011)

151. D. Inferior wall image

While it is difficult to entirely eliminate the attenuation of photon counts due to soft tissue, with single-photon emission computed tomography (SPECT), soft tissue attenuation can often be recognized and distinguished from true myocardial perfusion defects, thereby improving diagnostic accuracy.

(Hayes et al. 2003)

152. D. A soft tissue attenuation artifact

Abnormal function in conjunction with a similar fixed defect would be compatible with myocardial infarction or myocardial stunning.
(Zaret and Beller 2005)

153. D. MPI and initial troponin I values in samples drawn at the time of imaging have similar sensitivity for detection of acute MI

Initial troponin I values in samples drawn at the time of imaging have a sensitivity of only 39 %; reported SPECT sestamibi imaging performed in the emergency department was as high as 92 % sensitive for detection of acute MI. The maximum troponin I during the first 24 h had sensitivity similar to that of rest sestamibi imaging, but at a distinctly later time point.
(Wackers et al. 2002)

154. B. To perform exercise-induced stress MPI studies

N-13ammonia is a cyclotron product, and has a physical half-life of 9.96 min, allowing to perform exercise-induced MPI. Optimal PET imaging of the myocardium is generally achieved between 15 and 20 min after administration.
(Takalkar et al. 2011)

155. D. Necrosis

The ability to image cell death anywhere along the spectrum of apoptosis to necrosis allows investigators to apply a therapeutic regimen in the cardiovascular pathologies.
(Morrison and Sinusas 2009)

156. A. Directly proportional to the radiotracer concentration in the myocardium that matches that pixel

The comparative differences in count values between myocardial pixels are displayed in the images as a variation in either brightness (in black-and-white images) or color (in color images).
(Iskandrian and Garcia 2012)

157. C. <1 % per year

In the study by Machecourt et al, who followed up 1,926 patients for 33 months after exercise 201Tl-201 SPECT imaging, the cardiac mortality rate was 0.42 %/year in patients with normal scans and 2.1 %/year in patients with abnormal scans.
(Machecourt et al. 1994)

158. C. Fixed perfusion defects indicate a higher risk than ischemia for perioperative cardiac events

Fixed perfusion defects indicate a lower risk than ischemia for perioperative cardiac events; however, the risk is higher than that with a normal scan.
(Fleisher et al. 2007)

159. B. Soft tissue attenuation

   D. Abnormal lung uptake
   F. Patient motion
   The planar images provide valuable information about the proximity of soft tissue to the myocardial structures, as well as other incidental findings (e.g., neoplastic lesions).
   (Zaret and Beller 2005)

160. B. Recovery heart rate

   DTS = Exercise Time − (5 × Max ST) − (4 × Angina Index)
   (Mark et al. 1987)

161. B. Segmentation method

   In segmentation: the CT image is partitioned into regions of distinct tissue types, e.g., bone, soft tissue, and lung, and a fixed value that corresponds to the attenuation coefficient for the energy of the appropriate radionuclide is assigned to those regions.
   (Kinahan et al. 1998)

162. B. Integrins

   Integrins, which are members of a family of cell surface receptors, promote endothelial cell migration and survival during angiogenesis and lymphangiogenesis.
   (Morrison and Sinusas 2009)

163. A. Adenosine, regadenoson, and dipyridamole are equally effective in increasing coronary blood flow

   Adenosine, regadenoson, and dipyridamole are equally effective in increasing coronary blood flow, even though individual patients have significant variations in responses to these pharmaceuticals. The reported sensitivity and specificity for CAD diagnosis with dipyridamole and adenosine varies depending upon the definition of CAD and the prevalence of disease in the population studied.
   (Heller et al. Accessed July 22, 2011)

164. B. Rubidium underestimates myocardial flow at higher rates

   Like the SPECT tracers, Rb-82 also shows a plateau in myocardial extraction at hyperemic flows.
   (Ho and Reddy 2011)

165. B. Intercoronary steal

   Intercoronary steal occurs when the coronary bed distal to a severe stenosis is perfused with collaterals from another coronary artery territory. During vasodilatation, resistance in the normal coronary artery falls, resulting in increased flow in areas without stenosis, and reduced collateral flow to the region supplied by the stenotic artery segment
   (Akinboboye et al. 2001)

166. B. I-123 mIBG

Iobenguane, also known as metaiodobenzylguanidine or mIBG, or MIBG (Adreview), is a radiolabeled molecule similar to noradrenaline.
(Iskandrian and Garcia 2012)

167. A. Antianginal therapy with nitrates

Presences of left circumflex coronary artery stenosis, branch vessel or distal stenosis, and mild degree of stenosis (50–70 % luminal narrowing) also drop sensitivity of SPECT.
(Beller and Zaret 2000)

168. A. Apoptotic cells

Apoptosis occurs during acute cardiac allograft rejection and disappears after treatment of rejection. 99mTc-annexin V can be used to detect and monitor cardiac allograft rejection.
(Narula et al. 2004)

169. C. Direction of motion

The magnitude and timing of motion are the most important factors that influence whether image artifacts will arise; the direction and pattern of motion affect the location of these artifacts.
(Prigent et al. 1993)

170. C. 4.6 METs

Workloads are measured in metabolic equivalents (MET); 1 MET being the amount of oxygen consumed at bed rest (3.5 mL/kg/min).
(Bonow et al. 2011)

171. B. 50 % of peak LV intensity

RV uptake increases in the presence of RV hypertrophy, most frequently because of pulmonary hypertension.
(Wackers 2005)

172. A. Myocardial thickening

Parameters of diastolic function require a considerably greater number of gating intervals than are commonly exercised.
(Khalil 2011)

173. C. Sinus bradycardia with frequent PVCs

The term describes arrhythmias and conduction abnormalities that produce a heart rate of less than 60 beats/min. Sinus bradycardia always needs to be explained in clinical context because it may be a normal variant, e.g., in a healthy person during sleep or in a resting athlete, or may be due to drug effect/toxicity, e.g., beta blocker.
(Goldberger 2006)

174. C. Glutamine

The presence of ammonia N-13 and glutamine N-13 in the myocardium allows for PET imaging of the myocardium.
(Phelps 2004)

175. D. Scar tissue

LV end-diastolic wall thickness can be used as a marker of scar tissue.
(Schinkel et al. 2007)

176. A. 4–6 mSV

Radiation exposure to patients from cardiac: single isotope rest/stress thallium-201 imaging ~18–20 mSV, dual-isotope imaging (thallium and technetium) ~25–30 mSV, and single isotope rest/stress technetium imaging approximately 8–10 mSV.
(Cerqueira et al. 2010)

177. C. Tc-99m glucarate

Tc-99m glucarate activity continually and progressively increases in irreversibly injured myocardium, and its uptake is correlated with myocardial necrosis. Tc-99m glucarate did not accumulate in areas of ischemia and could be imaged in areas of infarction as early as 10 min post-reperfusion.
(Morrison and Sinusas 2009)

178. A. Amino acids

Cardiac amyloidosis, also known as "stiff heart syndrome," is the most typical form of restrictive cardiomyopathy, and may affect the heart conduction system that can lead to arrhythmias and conduction abnormalities. I-123MIBG imaging has shown marked cardiac sympathetic denervation, providing insight into the pathogenesis of cardiac conduction disturbances in amyloidosis.
(MedlinePlus Accessed September 22, 2012)

179. D. False positive studies

Filters that are too smooth may result in false negative studies, and filters that are too coarse may result in false positive studies.
(Cherry et al. 2003)

180. A. Anaerobic threshold

Although, a high correlation exists between a person's perceived exertion rating times 10 and the actual heart rate during physical activity, the Borg Rating of Perceived Exertion is also the preferred method to assess intensity among those individuals who take medications that affect heart rate or pulse.
(Bonow et al. 2011)

181. D. Increases at very low rates, decreases at very high flow rates

Tl-201 has a blood clearance half-time of <30 s and a first pass extraction in the myocardium of >85 %.
(Thrall and Taveras 2006)

182. D. 2.5 mL/min/g

The roll-off is the smallest for Tl-201 and is larger for Tc-99m sestamibi and Tc-99m tetrofosmin.
(Zaret and Beller 2005)

183. B. Correcting dual-isotope cross talk

Downscatter correction methods are not undoubted and have not been clinically substantiated.
(Husain 2007)

184. D. At flows of 2.5–3.0 mL/min/g, further flow increases are associated with progressively smaller increases in myocardial N-13 ammonia concentrations

Administered intravenously, nitrogen-13 (N-13) ammonia rapidly exchanges into the myocardium and clears from blood so that high contrast myocardial perfusion images are obtained within 5–15 min after the tracer administration.
(Schelbert 2009)

185. A. Adenosine

Rates of blood flow, presumably mediated by adenosine, adjust the diameter of the pre-arteriolar and arteriolar vessels and, thus, their resistance to flow; as a result substrate delivery is constantly adjusted to match energy demand.
(Schelbert 2009)

186. D. Right ventricle

Right ventricular systolic function may be assessed by calculation of RVEF from gated cardiac blood-pool imaging, multigated acquisition (MUGA); however, more accurate evaluation may require a different technique, such as first-pass RNA.
(Society of Nuclear Medicine Procedure Guideline Accessed July 12, 2012)

187. A. Deterministic effects

Deterministic effects are due to radiation-induced cell death which may cause the death of the individual, depending on the organs exposed and the dose received.
(Lombardi 1999)

188. B. In-111 labeled antimyosin antibody

In-111 antimyosin is a monoclonal antibody that binds to cardiac myosin exposed upon cell death. The sensitivity of an antimyosin scan is approximately 95 %, and the specificity is only in the 50% range.
(Margazi et al. 2003)

189. B. The radiation from a radioactive source is monoenergetic gamma-rays and polychromatic X-ray from an X-ray tube

The flux of X-ray photons from a typical X-ray tube is much higher than a conventional sealed source used in TCT, CT images can be acquired on the order of seconds to a few minutes depending on the X-ray tube strength.
(Holly et al. 2010)

190. A. The first stage of the Standard Bruce Test protocol

The first two stages of the Modified Bruce Test are performed at a 1.7 mph and 0 % grade and 1.7 mph and 5 % grade.
(Hill and Timmis Accessed Nov 21, 2012)

191. D. Without left ventricle hypertrophy

MPI is a Class I indication for CAD detection when LVH is present on ECG according to ACC/AHA guidelines.
(Hendel et al. 2002)

192. D. 200 cts

Peak pixel activity in the LV for Tl-201 should exceed 100 cts. The quality of the reconstructed data is a direct reflection of the count rates measured on the raw data.
(ASNC Accessed June 17, 2012)

193. D. Wiener filter

Wiener and Metz filters are adaptive filters—they not only suppress noise but also prevent blurring and the smoothing of edges of objects; ideally they reduce noise without disproportionately lowering resolution.
(Christian et al. 2004)

194. B. O-15 water

The tracer is not accumulated in the myocardium and instead reaches equilibrium between extra- and intravascular compartments; as a result processing for blood pool subtraction is needed.
(Bengel et al. 2009)

195. D. Obstructive shock

Obstructive shock results from impedance of the great vessels or the heart itself, by an intrinsic or extrinsic obstruction. Obstructive shock has much in common with cardiogenic shock, and the two are frequently grouped together
(Cotran et al. 2005)

196. A. The heart shifts slightly superior, and the diaphragm is more inferior in the prone position

The use of prone imaging can improve inferior wall image quality. In the prone position, the distance between the diaphragm and the inferior wall of the left ventricle is increased.
(Hayes et al. 2003)

197. D. Optimization

Justification indicates that no practice resulting in exposure to ionizing radiation should be implemented unless it results in sufficient net benefit to exposed individuals or society to compensate the harm.
(ICRP 1991)

198. D. The T wave is a marker of myocardial ischemia

In rare cases, a T wave inverted at rest and becoming upright with exercise may be a marker for myocardial ischemia in a patient with documented CAD; however, it would necessitate confirmatory testing such as the parallel finding of a reversible myocardial perfusion defect.
(Goldberger 2006)

199. A. Is more likely to introduce image artifacts

Movement that happens when the heart is near to the detector is more likely to create image artifacts, because the corresponding projections have better spatial resolution and provide more information to the final reconstructed SPECT images.
(Ibrahim and DiFilippo 2006)

200. C. Collimator-detector response

The resolution recovery method models the collimator-detector response in order to correct for noise and resolution degradation, and include intrinsic system response and collimator-specific geometric response.
(DePuey 2012)

201. D. Stent without restenosis

CT shows the stent in the proximal LAD to be patent without relevant in-stent restenosis (ISR). Coronary CT imaging of coronary artery stents progressed as a reliable tool in the diagnostic workup of patients after coronary revascularization therapy.
(Storto et al. 2002)

202. C. The Layer of Maximum Count (LMC) method

   LMC method was developed to solve the problem of small hearts. In patients with small hearts, most of the currently available methods tend to underestimate the LV and overestimate the EF. Layer of Maximum Count method is a distinctive methodology that uses the prolate-spheroid geometry—axis of symmetry is longer than its other axes—to sample the myocardium.
   (Feng et al. 2002)

203. C. Summed Rest Score (SRS)

   Summed Rest Score (SRS) is the total segmental scores of rest images.
   (Fuster et al. 2007)

204. C. Volume-weighting and distance-weighting methods

   The volume-weighting approach is likely to misrepresent the defect location but offers an accurate assessment of the defect size; the distance-weighting method have a tendency to alter the defect size at the cost of improving the accuracy of the defect location—for this reasons it is not recommended to merely depend on a polar map without paying attention to tomographic slices.
   (Khalil 2011)

205. C. A selective A_{2A} agonist with low-level exercise

   The addition of low-level exercise to regadenoson is feasible, well tolerated, and associated with fewer side effects compared to a standard adenosine-supine protocol (AdenoSup).
   (Thomas et al. 2009)

206. A. Distal LCX

   Dominance refers to whether the posterior descending artery (PDA) begins from the RCA (right dominant), LCX (left dominant), or both (codominant).
   (Smuclovisky 2009)

207. B. The mid-diastolic phase of the cardiac cycle

   The acquisition is based on a prospective electrocardiogram (ECG)-triggered sequential axial acquisition mode in opposition to the standard retrospectively gated continuous helical acquisition. PGA allows up to 80 % reduction of the radiation dose (approximately 3 mSv), similar to a calcium score.
   (Smuclovisky 2009)

208. C. A percutaneous femoral artery approach

   A percutaneous brachial artery approach is occasionally employed in patients with severe peripheral vascular disease (PVD) or when the groin access is not possible or technically difficult.
   (Ho and Reddy 2011)

209. B. Erectile dysfunction

In male patients referred for MPI sexual function, questioning may be useful
to stratify risk in patients suspected to have coronary heart disease.
(Min et al. 2006)

210. B. LCx-100 % stenosis (Fig. 4.11)

Cardiac arteries and Lesion findings:
LAD–lesion on Mid LAD: 30 % stenosis 15 mm length, lesion on first Diag:
70 % stenosis 10 mm length.
LCx-lesion on Prox Cx: 100 % stenosis 25 mm length
(RCA-lesion on Prox RCA: 50 % stenosis 40 mm length, moderate collateral
flow from the Dist. RCA to the Dist. Cx- coronary angiogram of the RCA not
shown)

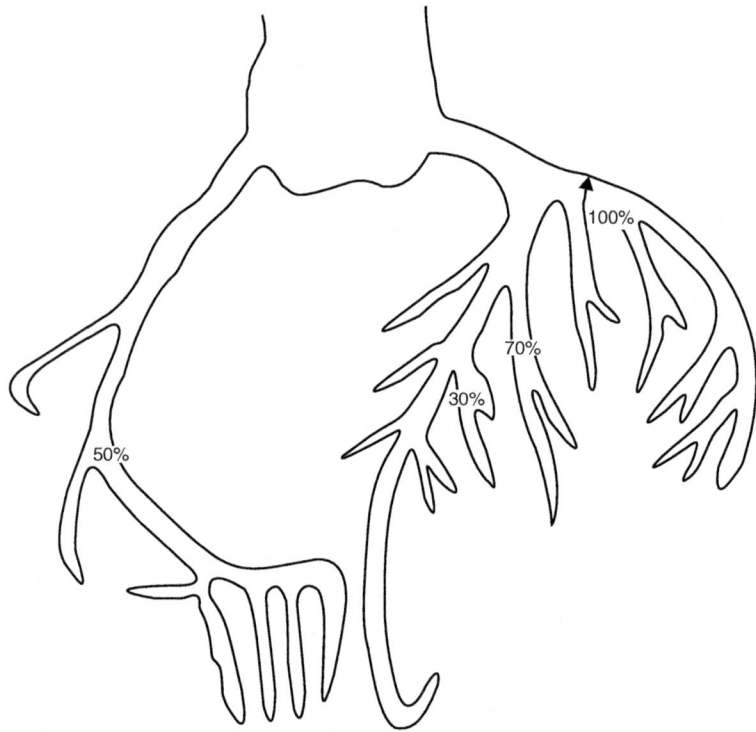

Fig. 4.11 Coronary tree

211. 20 % of that on the left

As the blood pressure on the right side is only approximately 20 % of that on the left, the RV has a much thinner muscular wall than the LV.
(Sharp et al. 2005)

212. B. Meiosis

Meiosis is a type of cell division that reduces the number of chromosomes in the parent cell by half and produces four gamete cells.
(Statkiewicz-Sherer et al. 2011)

213. C. LV ejection fraction is the strongest predictor of mortality

Perfusion defect reversibility is most predictive of future myocardial infarction; LV ejection fraction is the strongest predictor of mortality.
(Sharir et al. 2001)

214. D. Tracer selection

In patients with small LV cavities, the endocardial limits may be difficult to identify, and an underestimation of LV cavity size at end systole may lead to erroneously high LV ejection fraction values.
(Vallejo et al. 2000)

215. B. Atrial tachycardia

AT is a type of supraventricular tachycardia (SVT), which commences from a "focus" in either of the two top atrial chambers with a heart rate of >100 beats per minute.
(Walsh 2007)

References and Suggested Readings

ACC/AHA 2002 Guideline update for exercise testing: summary article. http://circ.ahajournals.org/cgi/content/full/106/14/1883.

Ahlberg AW, Baghdasarian SB, Athar H, et al. Symptom-limited exercise combined with dipyridamole stress: prognostic value in assessment of known or suspected coronary artery disease by use of gated SPECT imaging. J Nucl Cardiol. 2008;15:42.

Akinboboye OO, Idris O, Chou RL, et al. Absolute quantitation of coronary steal induced by intravenous dipyridamole. J Am Coll Cardiol. 2001;37:109.

Akinpelu D (ed). Treadmill stress testing. http://emedicine.medscape.com/article/1827089. Accessed 11 Oct 2012

Appropriate Use Criteria (AUC). http://www.astellasapps.com/web_app/resources-definitions.html. Accessed 12 June 2012

ASNC. http://www.asnc.org/imageuploads/ImagingGuidelinesFPRNA020509.pdf.

ASNC. Pharmacologic and exercise stress tests. http://www.asnc.org/media/PDFs/PPStressTests081511.pdf. Accessed 07 April 2012.

Astellas. http://www.astellas.us/docs/lexiscan.pdf . Accessed 28 July 2012

Baggish LA, Boucher AC. Radiopharmaceutical agents for myocardial perfusion imaging. Circulation. 2008;118:1668–74.

Banerjee A, Newman DR, Van den Bruel A, Heneghan C. Diagnostic accuracy of exercise stress testing for coronary artery disease: a systematic review and meta-analysis of prospective studies. Int J Clin Pract. 2012;66, 5:477–92.

Beller GA, Zaret BL. Contributions of nuclear cardiology to diagnosis and prognosis of patients with coronary artery disease. Circulation. 2000;101:1465.

Bengel MF, Higuchi T, et al. Cardiac positron emission tomography. J Am Coll Cardiol. 2009;54:1–15.

Biology on line. http://www.biology-online.org/dictionary/Ribosomes. Accessed 23 July 2012

Bogaty P, Poirier P, Boyer L, et al. What induces the warm-up ischemia/angina phenomenon: exercise or myocardial ischemia? Circulation. 2003;107:1858.

Bonow OR, Mann LD, Zipes PD, et al. Braunwald's heart disease—a textbook of cardiovascular medicine. 9th ed. Philadelphia: Elsevier Saunders; 2011.

Burrell S, MacDonald A. Artifacts and pitfalls in myocardial perfusion imaging. J Nucl Med Technol. 2006;34:193–211.

Bayes theorem. http://www.medterms.com/script/main/art.asp?articlekey=10301. Accessed 17 May 2012

Caldwell JH, Link JM, Levy WC, et al. Evidence for pre- to postsynaptic mismatch of the cardiac sympathetic nervous system in ischemic congestive heart failure. J Nucl Med. 2008;49(2):234–41.

CDC. Perceived exertion (Borg Rating of Perceived Exertion Scale). http://www.cdc.gov/physicalactivity/everyone/measuring/exertion.html. Accessed 20 Sept 2012

Cerqueira MD, Allman KC, Ficaro EP, et al. Recommendations for reducing radiation exposure in myocardial perfusion imaging. J Nucl Cardiol. 2010;17:709–18.

Cherry S, Sorenson J, Phelps M. Physics in nuclear medicine. 3rd ed. Philadelphia: Saunders; 2003.

Christian PE, Bernier DR, Langan JK. Nuclear medicine and PET. Technology and techniques. 5th ed. St. Louis, MO: Mosby; 2004.

Constantine G, Shan K, Flamm SD, Sivananthan MU. Role of MRI in clinical cardiology. Lancet. 2004;363:2162–71.

Cotran RS, Kumar V, Fausto N, et al. Robbins and Cotran pathologic basis of disease. St. Louis, MO: Elsevier Saunders; 2005.

DePuey EG. Advances in SPECT camera software and hardware: currently available and new on the horizon. J Nucl Cardiol. 2012;19(3):551–81.

Dilsizian V, Narula J, Braunwald E. Atlas of nuclear cardiology. 3rd ed. Philadelphia: Current Medicine; 2009.

Emmett L, Iwanochko RM, Freeman MR, Barolet A, Lee DS, Husain M. Reversible regional wall motion abnormalities on exercise technetium- 99m-gated cardiac single photon emission computed tomography predict high-grade angiographic stenoses. J Am Coll Cardiol. 2002;39:991–8.

English RJ, Brown SE. SPECT single photon emission computed tomography: a primer. 2nd ed. New York, NY: The Society of Nuclear Medicine; 1990.

Erlandsson K, Kacperski K, van Gramberg D, Hutton BF. Performance evaluation of D-SPECT: a novel SPECT system for nuclear cardiology. Phys Med Biol. 2009;54:2635.

Feng B, Sitek A, Gullberg GT. Calculation of the left ventricular ejection fraction without edge detection: application to small hearts. J Nucl Med. 2002;43:786–94.

Ficaro EP, Hansen CL. American Society of Nuclear Cardiology: Imaging guidelines for nuclear cardiology procedures. Available at: http://www.asnc.org/imageuploads/ImagingGuidelinesComplete070709.pdf. Accessed 01 June 2011.

Fleming JS. A technique for using CT images in attenuation correction and quantification in SPECT. Nucl Med Commun. 1989;10:83–97.

Fleisher LA, Beckman JA, Brown KA, et al. ACC/AHA 2007 guidelines on perioperative cardiovascular evaluation and care for noncardiac surgery: A report of the American College of Cardiology/American Heart Association Task Force on Practice Guidelines (Writing Committee to Revise the 2002 Guidelines on Perioperative Cardiovascular Evaluation for Noncardiac Surgery). J Am Coll Cardiol. 2007;50:e159.

Fukumoto M. Single-photon agents for tumor imaging: 201Tl, 99mTc- MIBI, and 99mTc-tetroformin. Ann Nucl Med. 2004;18:79–95.

Fuster V, O'Rourke RA, Walsh RA, Poole Wilson P. "Hurst's The Heart." 12th ed. 2007.

Germano G, Berman SD. Clinical gated cardiac SPECT. 2nd ed. Malden, MA: Blackwell; 2006.

Germano G. Technical aspects of myocardial SPECT imaging. J Nucl Med. 2001;42:1499–507.

Ghosh N, Rimoldi EO, Beanlands SBR, et al. Assessment of myocardial ischaemia and viability: role of positron emission tomography. Eur Heart J. 2010;31:2984–95.

Gibbons RJ, Balady GJ, Beasley JW, et al. ACC/AHA 2002 guideline update for exercise testing. Summary article. A report of the American College of Cardiology/American Heart Association Task Force on Practice Guidelines. Circulation. 2002;106(14):1883–92.

Gibbons RJ, Chatterjee K, Daley J, et al. ACC/AHA/ACP-ASIM guidelines for the management of patients with chronic stable angina: a report of the American College of Cardiology/American Heart Association Task Force on Practice Guidelines. J Am Coll Cardiol. 1999;33:2092–197.

Gibbons JR. Imaging techniques. Myocardial perfusion imaging. Heart. 2000;83:355–60.

Goldberger LA. Clinical electrocardiography: a simplified approach. 7th ed. St. Louis, MO: Mosby Elsevier; 2006.

Hayes SW, De Lorenzo A, Hachamovitch R, et al. Prognostic implications of combined prone and supine acquisitions in patients with equivocal or abnormal supine myocardial perfusion SPECT. J Nucl Med. 2003;44:1633.

Heller VG. Attenuation artifact in SPECT radionuclide myocardial perfusion imaging. http://www.uptodate.com/contents/attenuation-artifact-in-spect-radionuclide-myocardial-perfusion-imaging. Accessed 18 June 2012.

Heller VG, Lundbye BJ, Kapetanopoulos A. Vasodilator stress radionuclide myocardial perfusion imaging: testing methodologies and safety. http://www.uptodate.com. Accessed 22 July 2011.

Hendel CR et al. ACCF/ASNC/ACR/AHA/ASE/SCCT/SCMR/SNM 2009 appropriate use criteria for cardiac radionuclide imaging. J Am Coll Cardiol. 2009;53(23):2201–29.

Hendel RC, Corbett JR, Cullom SJ, et al. The value and practice of attenuation correction for myocardial perfusion SPECT imaging: a joint position statement from the American Society of Nuclear Cardiology and the Society of Nuclear Medicine. J Nucl Cardiol. 2002;9:135.

Hill J, Timmis A. ABC of clinical electrocardiography. Exercise tolerance testing. http://www.ncbi.nlm.nih.gov/pmc/articles/PMC1123032/pdf/1084.pdf. Accessed 21 Nov 2012.

Ho BV, Reddy PG. Cardiovascular imaging. St. Louis, Mo: Saunders Elsevier; 2011.

Holly AT, Abbott GB, Al-Mallah M, et al. ASNC imaging guidelines for nuclear cardiology procedures. Single photon-emission computed tomography. J Nucl Cardiol. 2010;17:941–73.

Husain SS. Myocardial perfusion imaging protocols: is there an ideal protocol? J Nucl Med Technol. 2007;35:3–9.

Ibrahim YD, DiFilippo PF. Optimal SPECT processing and display: making bad studies look good to get the right answer. J Nucl Cardiol. 2006;13:855–66.

ICRP. The 1996 ICRP21. Oxford: Pergamon; 1991.

ICRP 2001 Supporting Guidance 2. Radiation and your patient: a guide for medical practitioners. Ann ICRP 31. Pergamon, Oxford. ICRP website: www.icrp.org/docs/ICRP_85_Interventional_s.pps. Accessed 1 July 2012

Iskandar A, et al. Gender differences in the diagnostic accuracy of SPECT myocardial perfusion imaging: a bivariate meta-analysis. ASNC 2012

Iskandrian EA, Garcia VE. Atlas of nuclear cardiology: imaging companion to Braunwald's heart disease. Philadelphia, PA: Elsevier Saunders; 2012.

Iskandrian AE, Verani MS, et al. Nuclear cardiac imaging and principles applications. 3rd ed. New York: Oxford University Press; 2003.

Jaffer F, Narula J. Molecular imaging of atherosclerosis: a biologic roadmap. In: Dilsizian V, Narula J, Braunwald E, editors. Atlas of nuclear cardiology. 3rd ed. Philadelphia: Current Medicine; 2009.

Khalil MM, editor. Basic sciences of nuclear medicine. Berlin, Heidelberg: Springer; 2011.

Kinahan PE, Townsend DW, Beyer T, et al. Attenuation correction for a combined 3D PET/CT scanner. Med Phys. 1998;25:2046–53.

Klabunde ER. Cardiovascular physiology concepts. http://www.cvphysiology.com/CAD/CAD003. htm. Accessed 21 July 2012

Koller D. Assessing diagnostic performance in nuclear cardiology. J Nucl Cardiol. 2002;9:114–23.

Lombardi MH. Radiation safety in nuclear medicine. Boca Raton, FL: CRC Press LLC; 1999.

Martinez-Möller A, Souvatzoglou M, Navab N, et al. Artifacts from misaligned CT in cardiac perfusion PET/CT studies: frequency, effects, and potential solutions. J Nucl Med. 2007;48:188–93.

MacDonald A, Burrell AS. Infrequently performed studies in nuclear medicine: Part 1. J Nucl Med Technol. 2008;36:132–43.

Machecourt J, Longére P, Fagret D. Prognostic value of thallium-201 single-photon emission computed tomographic myocardial perfusion imaging according to extent of myocardial defect: study in 1,926 patients with follow-up at 33 months. J Am Coll Cardiol. 1994;23:1096–106.

Manglos SH, Thomas FD, Gagne GM, Hellwig BJ. Phantom study of breast tissue attenuation in myocardial imaging. J Nucl Med. 1993;34:992.

Margazi ZJ, Anastasiou-Nana MI, Terrovitis J, et al. Indium-111 monoclonal antimyosin cardiac scintigraphy in suspected acute myocarditis: evolution and diagnostic impact. Int J Cardiol. 2003;90:239.

Mark DB, Hlatky MA, Harrell Jr FE, Lee KL, Califf RM, Pryor DB. Exercise treadmill score for predicting prognosis in coronary artery disease. Ann Intern Med. 1987;106:793–800.

MedlinePlus. Cardiac amyloidosis. http://www.nlm.nih.gov/medlineplus/ency/article/000193. htm. Accessed 22 Sept 2012

Min KJ, Williams AK, Okwuosa MT, et al. Prediction of coronary heart disease by erectile dysfunction in men referred for nuclear stress testing. Arch Intern Med. 2006;166:201–6.

Morrison RA, Sinusas JA. New molecular imaging targets to characterize myocardial biology. Cardiol Clin. 2009;27:329–44.

Moyer AV; and on behalf of the U.S. Preventive Services Task Force Screening for Coronary Heart Disease with Electrocardiography: U.S. Preventive Services Task Force Recommendation Statement Ann Intern Med. 31 July 2012.

Narula J, Kietselaer B, Hofstra L. Role of molecular imaging in defining and denying death. J Nucl Cardiol. 2004;11:349.

O'Connor KM, Kemp JB. Single-photon emission computed tomography/computed tomography: basic instrumentation and innovations. Semin Nucl Med. 2006;36:258–66.

Papaioannou IG, Heller VG. Exercise radionuclide myocardial perfusion imaging in the diagnosis and prognosis of coronary heart disease. http://www.uptodate.com. Accessed 22 July 2011.

Paul KI, Nabi AH. Gated myocardial perfusion SPECT: basic principles, technical aspects, and clinical applications. J Nucl Med Technol. 2004;32:179–87.

Phelps ME, editor. PET: molecular imaging and its clinical applications. New York: Springer; 2004.

Prigent FM, Hyun M, Berman DS, Rozanski A. Effect of motion on thallium-201 SPECT studies: a simulation and clinical study. J Nucl Med. 1993;34:1845–50.

Rubidium Rb-82 Generator. http://www.nuclearonline.org/PI/Cardiogen.pdf. Accessed 13 July 2012.

Schelbert RH. Quantification of myocardial blood flow: what is the clinical role? Cardiol Clin. 2009;27:277–89.

Schinkel FLA, Poldermans D, Elhendy A, Bax JJ. Assessment of myocardial viability in patients with heart failure. J Nucl Med. 2007;48:1135–46.

Sharir T, Germano G, Kang XP, et al. Prediction of myocardial infarction versus cardiac death by gated myocardial perfusion SPECT: risk stratification by the amount of stress-induced ischemia and the poststress ejection fraction. J Nucl Med. 2001;42:831–7.

Sharir T, Germano G, Kavanagh PB, et al. Incremental prognostic value of poststress left ventricular ejection fraction and volume by gated myocardial perfusion single photon emission computed tomography. Circulation. 1999;100:1035–42.

Sharp FP, Gemmell GH, Murray DA, editors. Practical nuclear medicine. 3rd ed. Springer: London; 2005.

SNM.AHA.ACR. Standardization of cardiac tomographic imaging. J Nucl Med 33; 7 July 1992

Society of Nuclear Medicine. Procedure guideline for gated equilibrium radionuclide ventriculography. http://interactive.snm.org/docs/pg_ch01_0403.pdf. Accessed 12 July 2012

Smuclovisky C. Coronary artery CTA. A case based atlas. Heidelberg: Springer; 2009.

Statkiewicz-Sherer MA, Ritenour ER, Visconti PJ. Radiation protection in medical radiography. 6th ed. Maryland Heights, MO: Mosby Inc; 2011.

Storto LM, Marano R, Maddestra N, et al. Images in cardiovascular medicine. Multislice spiral computed tomography for in-stent restenosis. Circulation. 2002;105(16):2005.

Takalkar A, Agarwal A, Adams S, et al. Cardiac assessment with PET. PET Clin 2011;6(4)

Third Report of the National Cholesterol Education Program (NCEP) Expert Panel on Detection, Evaluation, and Treatment of High Blood Cholesterol in Adults (Adult Treatment Panel III) Final Report. Circulation 2002;106:3143.

Thomas GS, Thompson RC, Miyamoto MI, et al. The RegEx trial: a randomized, double-blind, placebo- and active-controlled pilot study combining regadenoson, a selective A $_{2A}$ adenosine agonist, with low-level exercise, in patients undergoing myocardial perfusion imaging. J Nucl Cardiol. 2009;16(1):63–72.

Thrall HJ, Taveras MJ. Nuclear medicine: the requisites in radiology. 3rd ed. Philadelphia, PA: Elsevier Mosby; 2006.

Toba M, Kumita S, Cho K, et al. Usefulness of gated myocardial perfusion SPECT imaging soon after exercise to identify postexercise stunning in patients with single-vessel coronary artery disease. J Nucl Cardiol. 2004;11:697–703.

Travin IM. Cardiac cameras. Semin Nucl Med. 2011;41:182–201.

Udelson JE, Shafer CD, Carrio I. Radionuclide imaging in heart failure: assessing etiology and outcomes and implications for management. J Nucl Cardiol. 2002;9:S40.

Vallejo E, Dione DP, Bruni WL, et al. Reproducibility and accuracy of gated SPECT for determination of left ventricular volumes and ejection fraction: experimental validation using MRI. J Nucl Med. 2000;41:874–82.

Voet D, Voet GJ, Pratt WC. Fundamentals of biochemistry. 2nd ed. Wiley. 2006.

Wackers FJT. On the bright side. J Nucl Cardiol. 2005;12:378–80.

Wackers FJT, Brown KA, Heller GV, et al. American Society of Nuclear Cardiology position statement on radionuclide imaging in patients with suspected acute ischemic syndromes in the emergency department or chest pain center. J Nucl Cardiol. 2002;9:246.

Wackers FJT, Bruni W, Zaret LB. Nuclear cardiology: the basics: how to set up and maintain a laboratory. Totowa, NJ: Humana; 2004.

Walsh EP. Interventional electrophysiology in patients with congenital heart disease. Circulation. 2007;115:3224–34.

Weber TK, Janicki SJ. The metabolic demand and oxygen supply of the heart: physiologic and clinical considerations. Am J Cardiol. 1979;44(4):1.

Wheat J, Currie G. Reconstruction strategies for gated myocardial perfusion SPECT: are false negatives a potential problem? Internet J Cardiol 2006; 4(1)

Yu CM, Lin H, Zhang Q, et al. High prevalence of left ventricular systolic and diastolic asynchrony in patients with congestive heart failure and normal QRS duration. Heart. 2003;89:54–60.

Zaidi H, Hasegawa B. Determination of the attenuation map in emission tomography. J Nucl Med. 2003;44:291.

Zaret BL, Beller GA. Clinical nuclear cardiology: state of the art and future directions. 3rd ed. Philadelphia, PA: Mosby; 2005.

Zubal GI, Wisniewski G. Understanding Fourier space and filter selection. J Nucl Cardiol. 1997;4:234–43.

Appendix A
Commonly Used Abbreviations and Symbols in Nuclear Medicine

Decay mode column

α	α decay
β⁻	β⁻ decay
ε	Electron Capture
β⁺	β⁺ decay
SF	Spontaneous Fission
β⁻β⁻	Double B⁻ Decay
β⁺β⁺	Double B⁺ Decay
IT	Isomeric Transition
p	Proton Emission
n	Neutron Emission
2D	Two-dimensional
2DE	Two-dimensional echocardiogram, echocardiography
3D	Three-dimensional
AAA	Abdominal aortic aneurysm
ABC	Airway, breathing, circulation
ABG	Arterial blood gases
ABW	Adjusted body weight
AC	Attenuation corrected
ACC	American College of Cardiology
ACE	Angiotensin converting enzyme
ACLS	Advance Cardiac Life Support
ACR	American College of Radiology
ACS	Acute Coronary Syndrome
AED	Automated external defibrillator
AF	Atrial fibrillation
AFL	Atrial flutter
AHA	American Heart Association

A. Moniuszko and B.A. Kesala, *Nuclear Cardiology Study Guide: A Technologist's Review for Passing Specialty Certification Exams*, DOI 10.1007/978-1-4614-8645-9, © Springer Science+Business Media New York 2014

AIPES	Association of Imaging Producers and Equipment Suppliers
AICD	Automatic implantable cardiac defibrillator
ALS	Advance Life Support
AMA	Against Medical Advice
AMI	Acute myocardial infarction
	Anterior myocardial infarction
Angio.	Angiogram
	Angiography
ANSI	American National Standards Institute
AO	Aorta
APC	Atrial premature contraction
AR	Aortic regurgitation
ARB	Angiotensin receptor blocker
ARF	Acute renal failure
ASA	Acetylsalicylic Acid (Aspirin)
ASNC	American Society of Nuclear Cardiology
ASTM	American Standards for Testing and Materials
AT	Atrial tachycardia
AUC	Appropriate use criteria
AV	Arteriovenous
A-V	Arterioventricular
AVM	Arteriovenous malformation
AVNRT	Atrioventricular nodal reentry tachycardia
AVR	Aortic valve replacement
BBB	Bundle branch block
BBB	Blood–brain barrier
BF	Blood flow
BG	Blood glucose
BLS	Basic Life Support
BMI	Body Mass Index
BMIPP	β-Methyl-p-[123I]iodophenyl–pentadecanoic acid
BNP	B-type natriuretic peptide
BP	Blood pressure
Bpm	Beats per minute
BRADY	Bradycardia
BSA	Body surface area
CABG	Coronary artery bypass graft
CAC	Coronary artery calcium
CACS	Coronary Artery Calcium Score
CAD	Coronary artery disease
CAFU	CArdiac FUnction
CAT	Computed axial tomography
Cath	Catheterization
CCT	Cardiac Computed Tomography
CCTA	Cardiac Computed Tomographic Angiography

CDR	Collimator detector response
CE	Cardiac enzymes
	Cardiac events
CFR	Coronary flow reserve
	Code of Federal Regulations
CGS	Centimeter–gram–second system
CHEER	Chest pain evaluation in the emergency room
CHF	Congestive heart failure
Chol	Cholesterol
CI	Cardiac Index
CK-MB	Creatine kinase-myocardial band
CM	Cardiomyopathy
CMR	Cardiac magnetic resonance
CMS	Centers for Medicare and Medicaid Services
CO	Cardiac output
CO_2	Carbon dioxide
COPD	Chronic obstructive pulmonary disease
CP	Chest pain
CPR	Cardiopulmonary resuscitation
CPT	Current procedural terminology
CRF	Chronic renal failure
CRP	C-Reactive Protein
CRT	Cardiac resynchronization therapy
	Coronary revascularization therapy
CSI	Cesium iodide
CTA	Computed tomography angiogram
CTDI	CT Dose Index
CVA	Cerebrovascular accident
CVD	Cardiovascular disease
CZT	Cadmium-zinc-telluride
D/C	Discharge
DCA	Digital cardiac angiography
DCM	Dilated cardiomyopathy
DDDR	Dual-chamber rate-adaptive pacemaker
DM	Diabetes mellitus
DMF	Drug master file
DNA	Deoxyribonucleic acid
DNR	Do not resuscitate
DOA	Dead on arrival
DOE	Dyspnea on exertion
DR	Digital radiography
DSP	Deconvolution of septal penetration
DTS	Duke Treadmill Score
DVT	Deep venous thrombosis
Dx	Diagnosis

e.g.	For example
E. S.R.D.	End stage renal disease
Ea.	Each
EBCT	Electron beam computed tomography
ECF	Extra cardiac findings
ECG	Electrocardiogram
ECT	Emory cardiac toolbox
ED	End diastole
EF	Ejection fraction
EMB	Endomyocardial biopsy
EMR	Electronic medical records
EP	Electrophysiology
EPS	Electrophysiologic study
Eq	Equal
ERASE	Emergency room assessment of Sestamibi for evaluation of chest pain
ERNA	Equilibrium radionuclide angiography
ES	End systole
ESR	Erythocyte sedimentation rate
et	And
ET	Emory toolbox
Etc	Et cetera
ETT	Exercise tolerance test
Eval	Evaluation
Excl.	Exclude
Exp.	Expired
Extr.	Extremities
FAO	Fatty acid oxidation
FBP	Filtered back projection
FBS	Fasting blood sugar
FDA	Food and drug administration
FDG	FluoroDeoxyGlucose
FFA	Free fatty acids
FFR	Fractional flow reserve
F-MISO	fluoromisonidazole
FN	False negative
FORE	Fourier rebinning
FOV	Field of view
FP	False positive
FPRNA	First-pass radionuclide angiography
f/u	Follow up
GCS	Glasgow coma scale
GEF	Global ejection fraction
GERD	GastroEsophageal reflux disease
GFR	Glomerular filtration rate
GLU	Glucose

Gm	Gram
GRAE	Generally regarded as effective.
GRAS	Generally regarded as safe
gSPECT	Gated single photon emission computed tomography
GSCQ	Gated SPECT cardiac quantification
G-tube	Gastrostomy tube
HAP	Hospital acquired pneumonia
Hb	Hemoglobin
HbA1c	Glycosylated hemoglobin
HCFA	Health Care Financing Administration
HCG	Human chorionic gonadotropin
HCM	Hypertrophic cardiomyopathy
Hct	Hematocrit
HCTZ	Hydrochlorothiazide
HD	High definition
HDL	High density lipoprotein
HF	Heart failure
H/H	Hemoglobin/Hematocrit
HLA	Horizontal long axis
HLTx	Heart and lung transplant
HLW	High-level waste
H/M	Heart-to-mediastinum ratio
HMO	Health maintenance organization
H/O	History of
H&P	History and physical
HR	Heart rate
HRCT	High-resolution CT
HRES	High resolution
HRR	Heart rate recovery
HRT	Hormone replacement therapy
HTN	Hypertension
HV	High voltage
IABP	Intra-aortic balloon pump
IAEA	International Atomic Energy Agency
IBW	Ideal body weight
IBP	Intraaortic balloon pump
ICA	Internal carotid artery
ICCU	Intensive Coronary Care Unit
ICD	Implantable cardioverter defibrillator
ICD-9	International classification of diseases (9th revision)
ICM	Ischemic cardiomyopathy
ICRP	International Commission on Radiological Protection
ICU	Intensive care unit
IDDM	Insulin dependent diabetes mellitus
IHD	Ischemic heart disease

IMACS	Image (management) archiving and communications system
IMP	IodoaMPhetamine
Inc	Incontinent
INF	Inferior
Inj	Injection
Insuff	Insufficiency
INT	Interior
I/O	Intake and output
ISO	International Standards Organization
ISR	In-stent restenosis
IV	IntraVenous(ly)
IVC	Inferior vena cava
IVCD	Interventricular conduction delay
JCAHO	Joint Commission on Accreditation of Healthcare Organizations
JPEG	Joint Photographic Experts Group
k	Kilo
K	Thousand
Kcal	Kilocalories
Kerma	Kinetic energy released in media
keV	Kiloelectron Volts
kg	Kilogram
L	Liter
LA	Left atrium
LAD	Left anterior descending coronary artery
	Left axis deviation
LAE	Left atrial enlargement
LAFB	Left anterior fascicular block
LAN	Local area network
LAO	Left anterior oblique
LBBB	Left bundle branch block
LCA	Left coronary artery
LCX	Left circumflex artery
LDL	Lower density lipoprotein
LE	Lower extremity
LFT	Liver function tests
L/H ratio	Lung-to-heart ratio
LIMA	Left internal mammary artery
LLAT	Left lateral
LLL	Left lower lobe
LLQ	Left lower quadrant
LMA	Left main artery
LMC	Layer of maximum count
LMP	Last menstrual period
LOR	Line of response
LPO	Left posterior Oblique

L-S	Lumbo-Sacral
LUE	Left upper extremity
LUL	Left upper lobe
LUQ	Left upper quadrant
LUT	Lookup table
LV	Left ventricle
LVEF	Left ventricle ejection fraction
LVG	Left ventriculography
LVGTF	left ventricular global thickening fraction
LVH	Left ventricular hypertrophy
LVOT	Left ventricular outflow tract
m	Meter
MACE	Major adverse cardiac events
MBF	Myocardial blood flow
MDCT	Muti-row detector CT scanner
mEq	MilliEquivalent
MET	Metabolic equivalent of task
MFR/3	Mean filling fraction
mg	Milligram
MHR	Multiple head registration
MI	Myocardial infarction
MIBG	MetaIodoBenzylGuanidine
MIRD	Medical internal radiation dose
MIP	Maximum intensity projection
μg	Microgram
MIP	Maximum intensity projection
ml	Milliliter
MLEM	Maximum likelihood expectation maximization
M&M	Morbidity and mortality
MPI	Myocardial perfusion imaging
MPR	Multiplanar reconstruction
MR	Mitral regurgitation
MRA	Magnetic resonance angiography
MRI	Magnetic resonance imaging
MRSA	Methicillin-resistant *Staphylococcus aureus*
MSAD	Multiple slice average dose
ms	Millisecond(s)
MUGA	Multi gated acquisition scan
MV	Mitral valve
MVO_2	Myocardial oxygen consumption
MVP	Mitral valve prolapse
MVR	Mitral valve replacement
N/A	Non applicable
NaCl	Sodium chloride
NAC	Non-attenuation corrected

NC	Nasal Cannula
NDA	New drug application
NECR	Noise Equivalent Count Rate
NEMA	National Electrical Manufacturers Association
NHLBI	National Heart, Lung and Blood Institute
ng	Nanogram(s)
NIDDM	Non-insulin dependent diabetes mellitus
NIH	National Institutes of Health
NIST	National Institute of Standards and Technology
NKA	No known allergies
Non-AC	Non-attenuation-corrected
NPO	Nothing per Oral
NRC	Nuclear Regulatory Commission
NSTEMI	Non-ST-segment elevation myocardial infarction
NSR	Normal sinus rhythm
NSVT	Nonsustained ventricular tachycardia
NYHA	New York Heart Association
OASIS	Organization to assess strategies for ischemic syndromes
OM	Obtuse marginal branch
OOB	Out of bed
OSEM	Ordered subsets expectation maximization
OP-OSEM	Ordinary Poisson OSEM
AW-OSEM	Attenuation-weighted OSEM
OSHA	Occupational Safety and Health Administration
OTC	Over the counter
p	After
P	P wave
PA	Pulmonary artery
PAC	Premature atrial contraction
PACS	Picture archiving and communication systems
PCD	Programmed cell death
PCI	Percutaneous coronary intervention
PCP	Primary care provider
PCWP	Pulmonary capillary wedge pressure
PDA	Patent ductus arteriosus
	Posterior descending coronary artery
PE	Pulmonary embolism
PEG	Percutaneous endoscopic gastrostomy
PET	Positron emission tomography
PET/CT	Positron emission tomography/computed tomography
PFR	Peak to filling rate
PFT	Pulmonary function tests
PGA	Prospectively gated axial
PH	Pulmonary hypertension
pH	Degree of acidity or alkalinity
PICC	Peripherally inserted central catheter

PMH	Past medical history
PMT	Pacemaker-mediated tachycardia
PN	Parenteral nutrition
PND	Paroxysmal nocturnal dyspnea
PNS	Peripheral nervous system
PO	Per Os
PPE	Personal protective equipment
PRN	Pro re nata: as necessary, as needed
Prox	Proximal
PSRF	Point source response function
PTCA	Percutaneous transluminal coronary angioplasty
PVCs	Premature ventricular contractions
PVD	Peripheral vascular disease
PVE	Partial-volume effect
PYP	Pyrophosphate
q	Every
QUADRAS	Quality Assessment of Diagnostic Accuracy
QC	Quality control
QF	Quality factor
q.h.	Every hour
q.i.d.	Four times daily
QGS	Quantitative gated SPECT
QPS-QGS	Quantitative perfusion SPECT/Quantitative gated SPECT
QRS	QRS complex
QS	QS complex
QT	Q to T interval
RA	Right atrium
RAD	Right axis deviation
RADAR	RAdiation Dose Assessment Resource
RAE	Right atrial enlargement
RBFMs	Radioactive blood flow markers
ROC	Receiver-operator characteristic
RAO	Right anterior oblique
RBBB	Right bundle branch block
RCA	Right coronary artery
RECIST	Response Evaluation Criteria in Solid Tumors
RF	Renal failure
Rh	Rhesus blood factor
RIS	Radioimmunoscintigraphy
RLAT	Right lateral
RLE	Right lower extremity
RLL	Right lower lobe
RLQ	Right lower quadrant
RLS	Restless leg syndrome
RMSSH	Rotating multi-segment slant-hole
RN	Registered nurse

RNA	Radionuclide angiography
RNA	Ribonucleic acid
ROI	Region of interest
R/O	Rule out
ROM	Range of motion
RP	RadioPharmaceutical
RR	Respiratory rate
RRNR	Resolution recovery-noise reduction
RUE	Right upper extremity
RUL	Right upper lobe
RUQ	Right upper quadrant
RV	Right ventricle
RVH	Right ventricular hypertrophy
RVOT	Right ventricular outflow tract
RWM	Regional wall motion
Rx	Prescription
SA	SinoAtrial
	Short axis
SB	Sinus Bradycardia
SCA	Sudden Cardiac Arrest
SCD	Sudden cardiac death
SD	Standard deviation
SDS	Summed Difference (stress-rest perfusion) Score
SICU	Surgical intensive care unit
SNR	Signal to noise ratio
SOAP	A standardized method for recording patient progress notes: S—subjective patient complaint, O—objective findings, A—assessment of the program, P—plan of action
SOB	Short of breath
S/P	Status post
SPECT	Single Photon Emission Computed Tomography
SRS	Summed Rest Score
S and S	Signs and symptoms
SSS	Summed Stress Score
SSS	Sick sinus syndrome
ST	Sinus tachycardia
ST	ST Segment
Stat	Immediately
STEMI	ST-segment elevation myocardial infarction
sTPD	Total perfusion deficit at stress
Sup	Supine
SV	Stroke volume
SVC	Superior vena cava
SVG	Saphenous vein graft
SVT	Supraventricular Tachycardia
SVR	Systemic vascular resistance

SWT	Systolic wall thickening
T	T Wave
TAC	Time–activity curve
TCP/IP	Transmission Control Protocol/Internet Protocol
TCR	Transmission-to-cross-talk ratio
TDD	Telecommunications device for the deaf
TED	Thrombo embolic deterrent (Ted stockings)
TEE	Transesophageal echocardiogram
TET	Treadmill exercise testing
THR	Target heart rate
TIA	Transient ischemic attack
TID	Transient ischemic dilation
t.i.d.	Three times a day
TIFF	Tagged image file format
TIMI	Thrombolysis in myocardial infarction
TN	True negative
TP	True positive
TPN	Total parenteral nutrition
TPR	Temperature, pulse, respiration
TTE	TransThoracic echocardiography
TTFR	Time to peak filling rate
TV	Tricuspid valve
UA	Unstable angina
UA/NSTEMI	Unstable angina and non-ST-elevation myocardial infarction
VANQWISH	Veterans' Affairs non-Q wave infarction strategies in hospital
VEGF	Vascular endothelial growth factor
VEGFRs	Vascular endothelial growth factor receptors
VF SCA	Ventricular fibrillation sudden cardiac arrest
via	By way of
VLA	Vertical long-axis
VLDL	Very low-density lipoprotein
VMA	Vanillymandelic acid
VOI	Volume of interest
V-P shunt	Ventriculo-peritoneal shunt
VRT	Volume rendered techniques
VS	Vital signs
VSD	Ventricular septal defect
VT	Ventricular tachycardia
VVI	Ventricular demand inhibited pacemaker
V-tach	Ventricular Tachycardia
WLCQ	Wackers-Liu Circumferential Quantification
WMSI	Wall motion score index
WMAs	Wall motion/thickening abnormalities
WPW	Wolff-Parkinson-White syndrome
YTD	Year to Date

Symbols

&	And
@	At
$\sqrt{}$	Check
$\downarrow$	Decrease
=	Equal
♀	Female
←	From
>	Greater Than
↑	High
↑	Increased
+++	Large Amount
<	Less Than
$\downarrow$	Low
$\downarrow$	Decreased
♂	Male
++	Moderate Amount
+	More or Less
-	Negative
O	No; Null; None; Nothing
#	Number
O	Objective Findings
+	Positive
1°	Primary
(?)	Questionable
2nd	Secondary; Second
2°	Secondary to
2°	Second Degree
ĉ	With
ŝ	Without

References

Hamilton B, Guidos B. Medical acronyms, symbols, and abbreviations. 2nd ed. New York, NY: Neal-Schumann; 1988.

Jablonski S. Dictionary of medical acronyms and abbreviations. Philadelphia, PA: Hanley and Belfus; 1987.

Logan CM, Rice MK. Logan's medical and scientific abbreviations. Philadelphia, PA: Lippincott; 1987.

Mosby's medical, nursing, and allied health dictionary. 3rd ed. St Louis, Mo: Mosby–Year Book, 1990

Webster JG. Encyclopedia of medical devices and instrumentation, vol. 1–4. Wiley: New York, NY; 1988.

Appendix B
Glossary of Cardiology Terms

Ablation The therapeutic removal, isolation, or destruction of cardiac tissue or conduction pathways involved in arrhythmias. Most often, cardiac ablation is used to treat rapid heartbeats that begin in the upper chambers (atria) or in the atrioventricular (AV) node.

Adenosine Naturally occurring substance produced in many sites in the body that plays a role in important biochemical processes. It can cause dilation of coronary arteries, as well as many other effects, e.g., regulating heart rhythm, toning blood vessels.

Aerobic respiration A form of cellular respiration that requires oxygen in order to generate energy

Algorithm A set of precise rules or procedures programmed into a pacemaker or defibrillator that are designed to solve a specific problem.

Alpha blockers A group of drugs used to lower blood pressure by blocking the effects of certain chemicals or hormones (specifically adrenaline or adrenaline-like substances) on alpha receptors.

Amiodarone A Class III antiarrhythmic drug (potassium channel blocker) used to slow the heart rate and help keep it in a regular rhythm. Side effects are usually dose related, and regular follow-up is necessary to determine kidney, liver, and lung function.

Aneurysm An abnormal widening or ballooning out of the wall of an artery, a vein, or the heart due to weakening of the wall by disease, injury, or an abnormality present at birth.

Angina pectoris (Angina) Medical term for chest pain or discomfort due to coronary heart disease. It occurs when the heart muscle (myocardium) doesn't get as much blood (hence as much oxygen) as it needs for a given level of work.

Angiogenesis Is the physiological process involving the growth of new blood vessels from preexisting vessels. The body creates small blood vessels called "collaterals" to help compensate for reduced blood flow.

A. Moniuszko and B.A. Kesala, *Nuclear Cardiology Study Guide: A Technologist's Review for Passing Specialty Certification Exams*, DOI 10.1007/978-1-4614-8645-9, © Springer Science+Business Media New York 2014

Angiography An X-ray test used to detect and diagnose diseases of the blood vessels and to examine the chambers of the heart. The X-ray is taken after the vessels have been injected with a dye that allows them to be visualized (angiogram).

Angioplasty A medical procedure in which a balloon is used to open narrowed or blocked coronary arteries. A catheter with a deflated balloon on its tip is passed into the narrowed artery segment, the balloon is inflated, and the narrowed segment widened. Then the balloon is deflated and the catheter is removed.

Angiotensin A chemical produced by the body that acts as a vasoconstrictor, causing the muscles around the blood vessels to contract, thus narrowing the blood vessels.

Angiotensin-Converting Enzyme (ACE) Inhibitors A class of drugs used to treat high blood pressure and heart failure. ACE inhibitors stop the body's production of angiotensin, which lowers blood pressure, increases blood flow to the heart, and reduces the heart's workload. Common ACE inhibitors are captopril, enalapril, lisinopril, and ramipril.

Angiotensin II receptor blockers (or Inhibitors) (ARBs) A class of drugs used to treat high blood pressure and heart failure. They do not interfere with the body's production of angiotensin. They block the effects of angiotensin, preventing it from constricting the muscles around the blood vessels, and narrowing the blood vessels. Common Angiotensin II Receptor Blockers (or Inhibitors) (ARBs) are valsartan, losartan, and olmesartan.

Antiarrhythmic medication A group of drugs that helps control and slow heart rate. They do this by either suppressing (slowing) the activity of tissue that is initiating electrical impulses too quickly in the heart's natural pacemaker (the sinoatrial or SA node) or by slowing the transmission of fast electrical impulses inside the heart.

Anticoagulants (Blood thinners) A group of drugs that decrease the ability of the blood to clot or coagulate. They are given to certain people at high risk for forming blood clots, such as those with artificial heart valves, or who have atrial fibrillation. Anticoagulants do not dissolve clots, but may prevent existing clots from becoming larger and causing more serious problems, and are often prescribed to prevent first or recurrent heart attack or stroke. Common anticoagulant drugs are heparin and warfarin.

Antihypertensive drugs a group of drugs commonly prescribed to help lower blood pressure when appropriate diet and regular physical activity alone have not succeeded. They include diuretics, angiotensin-converting enzyme (ACE) inhibitors, angiotensin receptor blocker (ARBs), vasodilators, alpha-blockers, beta-blockers, calcium channel blockers, and central alpha-agonists.

Antiplatelet agents A group of drugs used to keep blood clots from forming by preventing blood platelets from sticking together. They help prevent clotting in patients who have had a heart attack, unstable angina, ischemic strokes, transient ischemic attacks, (TIA,) and other forms of cardiovascular disease. Aspirin and clopidogrel are examples.

Aorta The large artery that receives blood from the heart's left ventricle and distributes it to the body.

Aortic stenosis (AS) A congenital heart defect in which the aortic valve, between the left ventricle and the aorta, is narrowed. The major symptoms of aortic stenosis are: chest pain, syncope, and shortness of breath (due to heart failure).

Aortic valve The heart valve between the left ventricle and the aorta. It has three flaps (cusps).

Arrhythmia (Dysrhythmia) An irregular heartbeat—the heart may beat too fast (tachycardia), too slowly (bradycardia), too early (premature contraction). or too irregularly (fibrillation).

Arterioles Small, muscular branches of arteries. The greatest change in blood pressure and velocity of blood flow occurs at the transition of arterioles to capillaries.

Arteriosclerosis Hardening of the arteries, which includes a variety of conditions that cause artery walls to thicken and lose elasticity, e.g., fatty deposits on the inner lining of arteries, calcification of the wall of the arteries, or thickening of the muscular wall of the arteries from chronically elevated blood pressure. Atherosclerosis is a form of arteriosclerosis.

Artery One of a series of vessels that carry oxygenated blood from the heart to the various parts of the body.

Artificial heart A prosthetic device that is implanted into the body to replace the original biological heart.

Asystole An abnormal heart rhythm characterized by an absence of electrical activity. Because there is no electrical activity, there is no heartbeat. This condition is followed by death if not treated and reversed immediately.

Atherectomy A procedure to remove plaque from arteries.

Atherosclerosis A form of arteriosclerosis in which the inner layers of artery walls become thick and irregular due to deposits of fat, cholesterol, and other substances ("plaque").

Atria The upper two chambers of the heart, known as the right atrium and left atrium. The atria are separated from the ventricles by valves and from each other by the atrial septum. The right atrium collects deoxygenated blood from the body and passes it to the right ventricle. The left atrium collects oxygenated blood from the lungs and passes it to the left ventricle.

Atrial fibrillation (AF) An irregular and often rapid heart rate that commonly causes poor blood flow to the body. Blood that isn't pumped completely out of the atria when the heart beats may pool and clot. Since 15 % of strokes occur in people with atrial fibrillation, its treatment is important to stroke prevention.

Atrial flutter (AFL) Very rapid beating of the heart's atria. This rhythm occurs most often in people with heart diseases such as pericarditis, coronary artery disease, and cardiomyopathy. Atrial flutter is typically not a stable rhythm and often degenerates into atrial fibrillation.

Atrial tachycardia (AT) A rapid heart rate that starts in the atria (includes AF and AFL)

Atrioventricular (AV) Node One of the major elements in the cardiac conduction system, which generates electrical impulses, and conducts them throughout the muscle of the heart, stimulating the heart to contract and pump blood.

Atrioventricular (AV) synchrony The normal activation sequence of the heart in which the atria contract, and then, after a brief delay, the ventricles contract. Dual chamber pacemakers are designed to attempt to maintain AV synchrony.

Autograft A graft in which material is transferred from one part of a person's body to another part.

Base The upper part of the heart involving the left atrium, part of the right atrium, and the proximal portions of the great vessels

B-type natriuretic peptide (BNP) Is secreted by the ventricles of the heart in response to excessive stretching of heart muscle cells. The physiologic actions of BNP include decrease in systemic vascular resistance, central venous pressure, as well as an increase in natriuresis. Higher BNP levels correlate with worse degrees of heart failure.

Beta-blockers (Beta-adrenergic blocking agents) A class of drugs that slow the heartbeat, lessen the force with which the heart muscle contracts, and reduce blood vessel contraction in the heart, brain, and throughout the body. Beta-blockers are also used to treat high blood pressure and other heart conditions by reducing the heart rate and the heart's output of blood. Atenolol, propranolol, metaprolol, and esmolol are examples of beta blockers.

Bicuspid aortic valve A congenital heart defect in which the aortic valve (valve between the left ventricle and the aorta) has only two flaps (cusps or leaflets) instead of the normal three.

Blood clot The final product of the blood coagulation step in hemostasis. A blood clot in an artery is called an arterial thrombosis; in the vein it is called a venous thrombosis. When an arterial or venous thrombosis breaks loose and travels through the bloodstream, it is called an embolus.

Blood pressure The force or pressure exerted by the heart against the walls of the arteries. High blood pressure increases the risk for heart attack, angina, stroke, kidney failure, peripheral artery disease, and atherosclerosis. The risk of heart failure also increases due to the increased workload that high blood pressure places on the heart.

Blood vessel dilators (Vasodilators) Drugs that cause the blood vessels (especially the arterioles) to expand by relaxing their muscular walls. ACE inhibitors and nitroglycerine are examples of vasodilators.

Body mass index (BMI) A formula to assess a person's body weight relative to height. BMI is determined by weight in kilograms divided by height in meters squared (kg/m^2). In studies by the National Center for Health Statistics, BMI values less than 18.5 are considered underweight. Those from 18.5 to 24.9 are healthy. Overweight is defined as a body mass index of 25.0–29.9. A BMI of about 25 kg/m^2 corresponds to about 10 % over ideal body weight. Obesity is defined as a BMI of 30.0 or greater (based on criteria of the World Health Organization), or about 30 pounds overweight. People with a BMI of 30 or more are at high risk of cardiovascular disease. Extreme obesity is defined as a BMI of 40 or greater.

Bradycardia A heart rate that is abnormally slow; commonly defined as under 60 beats per minute, or a rate that is too slow to physiologically support a person and their activities. Bradycardia can be present in otherwise normal individuals and is common in well-trained athletes and in most persons during deep sleep. If it presents no symptoms, it usually doesn't require treatment.

Bundle of His Is located in the proximal intraventicular septum. It emerges from the AV node to begin the conduction of the impulse from the AV node to the ventricles.

Calcium channel blockers (Calcium Antagonists) A class of drugs that blocks the movement of calcium into the heart and blood vessel muscle cells. This causes the muscles to relax, lowering blood pressure, slowing the heart rate, and decreasing oxygen demands of the heart. Since they decrease the heart's pumping strength, slow the heart rate, and relax blood vessels, they are also used to treat other heart conditions, such as chest pain (angina) and abnormal heart rhythms (arrhythmias). Amlodipine, diltiazem, nifedipine, and verapamil are examples of calcium channel blockers.

Capillaries Microscopically small blood vessels between arteries and veins that distribute oxygenated blood to the body's tissues.

Cardiac arrest Failure of the heart to pump blood through the body. Most cardiac arrests occur when the electrical impulses in the diseased heart become rapid (ventricular tachycardia), chaotic (ventricular fibrillation), or both. Cardiac arrest can be reversed if it's treated within a few minutes with cardiopulmonary resuscitation (CPR) and an electric shock (defibrillation) to the heart to restore a normal heartbeat.

Cardiac catheterization Is a medical procedure used to diagnose and treat some heart conditions and involves passing a thin long tube called a catheter into the right or left side of the heart, usually from the groin or the arm. Angiography and angioplasty (PCI, Balloon Angioplasty) are done during a cardiac cath. Cardiac Computed Tomography (CT scan), Computerized Axial Tomographic Scan (CAT scan)—an X-ray imaging technique that uses a computer to produce tomographic, or cross-sectional, images of the chest (including the heart and great vessels) or the brain.

Cardiac enzymes Enzymes in the body that are sometimes called heart damage markers because they are released into the bloodstream when heart muscle cells are damaged. These include the enzymes creatine phosphokinase (CPK), creatine kinase (CK), and the proteins troponin I (TnI) and troponin T (TnT).

Cardiac Positron Emission Tomography (PET) A noninvasive nuclear imaging technique used to assess myocardial perfusion, left ventricular function, and viability by reflecting the distribution of radiotracers injected into the body. The most frequently used radiotracers include fluorine-18 fluorodeoxyglucose (FDG), rubidium-82 (Rb-82), and nitrogen-13 ammonia (N-13).

Cardiac rehabilitation Cardiovascular rehabilitation is a medically supervised program to help heart patients recover quickly and improve their overall physical and mental functioning. Research has shown that patients who participate in rehabilitation programs have a higher survival rate and a better quality of life.

Cardiac tamponade The pericardial sac fills with fluid for any number of reasons, resulting in constriction of heart function.

Cardiomyopathy The general term for diseases of the heart muscle. The most common of these diseases is the dilated cardiomyopathy in which the disease weakens the heart muscle and causes left ventricular dilation leading to increased diastolic pressure and volume.

Cardiomyoplasty An investigational procedure in which skeletal muscles are taken from a patient's back or abdomen and wrapped around an ailing heart. Recent research suggests that it may not be as effective as originally hoped.

Cardiopulmonary Bypass (Heart/Lung Machine) A procedure that involves diverting blood from the heart and lungs through a heart/lung machine and the return of oxygenated blood to the aorta.

Cardiopulmonary resuscitation (CPR) An emergency lifesaving procedure that is performed when a person's own breathing or heartbeat has stopped. It uses a combination of chest compressions and rescue breathing.

Cardiovascular Pertaining to the heart and blood vessels..

Cardioversion Delivering an electrical shock to a person's heart to rapidly restore an abnormal heart rhythm (arrhythmia) back to normal. External cardioversion is performed with a defibrillator, either in an emergency situation, or as a scheduled treatment for arrhythmia. Internal cardioversion is delivered by a device similar to a pacemaker, called an implantable cardioverter defibrillator (ICD).

Cholesterol A soft, waxy substance found among the lipids in the bloodstream and in all the body's cells. It's an important part of a healthy body because it's used to form cell membranes, some hormones, and is needed for other functions. Cholesterol and other fats can't dissolve in the blood. They have to be transported to and from the cells by special carriers called lipoproteins.

Cholesterol-lowering drugs Cholesterol-lowering drugs reduce LDL ("bad") cholesterol, increase HDL ("good") cholesterol, and reduce triglycerides (a blood fat) depending on the class of drugs. Due to potential side effects, patients who are taking most cholesterol-lowering drugs may need to have periodic liver function tests. Several classes of drugs are used to treat cholesterol including statins.

Chordate Tendons that hold the valve flaps taunt, preventing backflow when the heart contracts

Chronotropic incompetence The inability of the heart to increase its rate appropriately in response to increased activity or metabolic need, e.g., exercise, illness, etc.

Claudication Pain caused by too little blood flow during exercise and generally affects the blood vessels in the legs. It is a common, early symptom of peripheral artery disease (PAD). Sometimes is called intermittent claudication.

Coarctation of the aorta A congenital heart defect (birth defect), in which the major artery from the heart (aorta) is narrowed (constricted) somewhere along its length. This obstructs blood flow to the lower part of the body and increases blood pressure above the constriction.

Collateral circulation The process in which a system of small normally closed arteries opens up and starts to carry blood to parts of the heart when a coronary artery is blocked. They can serve as alternate routes of blood supply.

Congenital heart disease (CHD) A broad term for a number of different abnormalities present at birth (congenital) affecting the heart. Congenital heart disease is often divided into two types: those with cyanosis (blue discoloration caused by a relative lack of oxygen) and those without cyanosis.

Congestive heart failure (Heart Failure) Congestive heart failure is a subcategory of heart failure when excess fluid, such as in the lungs or extremities, is present. Systolic dysfunction (or systolic heart failure) occurs when the heart muscle doesn't contract with enough force, so there is less oxygen-rich blood that is pumped throughout the body. Diastolic dysfunction (or diastolic heart failure) occurs when the heart contracts normally, but the ventricles do not relax properly or are stiff, and less blood enters the heart during normal filling.

Coronary arteries The two coronary arteries originate as the right and left main coronary arteries, which exit the ascending aorta just above the aortic valve, then arch down over the top of the heart and branch out in additional arteries that provide blood to the heart muscle.

Coronary artery bypass graft (Bypass surgery) Surgery that reroutes (bypasses) blood around clogged coronary arteries and improves the supply of blood and oxygen to the heart muscle. It's sometimes called open-heart surgery or CABG (for coronary artery bypass graft) or "cabbage."

Coronary artery disease (CAD) Conditions that cause narrowing of the coronary arteries, reducing blood flow to the heart muscle.

Coronary occlusion (or coronary thrombosis) An obstruction of a coronary artery that hinders blood flow to some part of the heart muscle.

C-reactive protein (CRP) test Blood test that measures the concentration of C-reactive protein (CRP), a plasma protein known as acute phase protein, that rises in the blood with inflammation from certain conditions. Since inflammation is believed to play a role in the development of coronary artery disease (atherosclerosis), a highly sensitive assay (hs-CRP) test may be added to the screening battery of cholesterol and other lipid tests to help detect people at risk for a heart attack.

Creatinine Is a breakdown product of creatine phosphate generated from muscle metabolism. Creatinine is usually filtered out by the kidneys and leaves the body.

Cuspid The tissue flaps that make a valve. Bi- and tri-cuspid refer to the number of flaps (two and three).

Cyanosis A bluish discoloration of the skin or mucous membranes caused by lack of oxygen in the blood

Cyanosis A condition in which a person's skin is discolored to a bluish hue because of inadequate oxygenation of the blood

Defibrillation Termination of an erratic, life-threatening arrhythmia of the ventricles by a high energy, direct current delivered asynchronously to the cardiac tissue. The defibrillation discharge will often restore the heart's normal rhythm.

Defibrillator A device that delivers "pacing" or an electric shock to the heart when an abnormal rhythm (arrhythmia) is detected. External defibrillators use pads that are placed on the chest to deliver the electric shock. Internal defibrillators (implantable cardioverter defibrillators or ICDs) continuously monitor the heart rhythm to detect overly rapid arrhythmias, such as ventricular tachycardia or ventricular fibrillation, and deliver precisely calibrated and timed electrical shocks to restore a normal heartbeat .

Diastole Relaxation of the heart, allowing blood to flow into the atria and ventricles

Diastolic blood pressure The lowest blood pressure measured in the arteries that occurs when the heart muscle relaxes between beats. In a typical blood pressure reading, such as 120/80, the lower number is diastolic blood pressure.

Diastolic dysfunction Abnormal function of the heart during its relaxation phase due to thickening (hypertrophy), cardiomyopathy, or due to stiffening of the sac around the heart (pericardium)

Diastolic heart failure A condition in which the pumping chambers (ventricles) of the heart become thickened, grow stiff, and cannot relax enough to adequately fill the heart's lower chambers (ventricles) with blood. The fluid then backs up into organs and causes edema and congestion even.

Digital cardiac angiography (DCA) A modified form of computer imaging that records pictures of the major blood vessels to the heart or brain

Digitalis The use of Digitalis purpurea extract containing cardiac glycosides for the treatment of heart conditions was first described in the English-speaking medical literature by William Withering, in 1785, which is considered the beginning of modern therapeutics. The American College of Cardiology and the American Heart Association guidelines recommend digoxin for symptomatic chronic heart failure for patients with reduced systolic function, preservation of systolic function, and/or rate control for atrial fibrillation with a rapid ventricular response. Digoxin , Digitoxin, Lanoxicaps, and Lanoxin are digitalis.

Diuretics (or Water Pills) Drugs that increases the rate at which urine forms by promoting the excretion of water and salts, help to relieve the heart's workload ,and also decreases the build up of fluid in the lungs and other parts of the body. Chlorothiazide, hydrochlorothiazide, and furosemide are examples of diuretics.

Dual-chamber pacemaker A pacemaker with two leads (one in the atrium and one in the ventricle) to allow pacing and/or sensing in both chambers of the heart to artificially restore the natural contraction sequence of the heart (physiologic pacing).

Dyspnea Difficulty in breathing often caused by heart conditions. Dyspnea on exertion (DOE) is the shortness of breath that occurs with increasing activity. Paroxysmal nocturnal dyspnea (PND) is a shortness of breath that awakens a person at night from sleep.

Echocardiography (Echocardiogram) A diagnostic method in which a hand-held device is placed on the chest, and high-frequency sound waves (ultrasound) are used to produce images of the heart's size, structure, and motion. Transthoracic echocardiogram (TTE) is the type of echocardiogram that most people will have a transducer that releases high-frequency sound waves is placed on the ribs near the breast bone and directed toward the heart.

Transesophageal echocardiogram (TEE) A scope is inserted down the patient's throat and it is used to get a clearer echocardiogram of the heart.

Edema Swelling due to an abnormally large amount of fluid in the intracellular body tissue spaces. Edema is common in the legs, ankles, and lungs of people with heart failure.

Ejection Fraction The proportion of the volume of blood in the ventricles at the end of diastole that is ejected during systole; it is the stroke volume divided by the end-diastolic volume, often expressed as a percentage.

Electrocardiogram (ECG) A printout from an electrocardiography machine used to measure and record the electrical activity of the heart.

Electromagnetic Interference (EMI) Equipment and appliances that use magnets and electricity have electromagnetic fields around them. If these fields are strong, they may interfere with the operation of the ICD.

Electrophysiology (EP) Study The use of programmed stimulation protocols to assess the electrical activity of the heart in order to diagnose arrhythmias.

Embolus A blood clot or other particle that forms in one part of the body, then moves through the bloodstream until it lodges in a narrowed vessel and blocks the flow of blood (circulation).

Endarterectomy Surgical removal of plaque deposits or blood clots in an artery.

Endocarditis An inflammation of the heart lining or valves, usually caused by bacterial infection. People with prosthetic heart valves, previous endocarditis, previous heart valve surgery, abnormal heart valves, or certain congenital heart defects are at increased risk of endocarditis.

Endocardium The innermost layer of endothelial tissue that lines the chambers of the heart.

Endothelium The smooth inner lining of some body structures, including the heart (endocardium) and blood vessels.

Epicardium The inner layer of the pericardium that is in actual contact with the surface of the heart. The epicardium contains the epicardial coronary arteries and veins, autonomic nerves, and lymphatic vessels.

Exercise stress test (Treadmill test) A diagnostic test in which a person walks on a treadmill or pedals a stationary bicycle while hooked up to equipment that monitors the heart. The test monitors heart rate, breathing, blood pressure, electrical activity (on an electrocardiogram), and the person's level of exhaustion (Exercise Test, Exercise Cardiac Stress Test or ECST).

Fibrillation A chaotic and unsynchronized quivering of the myocardium during which no effective pumping occurs. Fibrillation may occur in the atria or the ventricles.

Fourier transform A mathematical process that converts matrix information into frequency domain

Frame mode A method of computer data collection where x and y positional signals are stored in a single matrix.

Frequency The number of occurrences of a repeating event per unit time (temporal frequency).

Gray scale A continuous spectrum of shades of the color gray used to differentiate structures on a digital image.

Greenfield filter A type of inferior vena cava filter for use in the prevention of clot propagation to the lungs.

HDL Cholesterol (High-Density Lipoprotein Cholesterol) Often called "good" cholesterol because a high level of it protects against heart attack and other cardiovascular conditions. People with a low HDL cholesterol level (less than 40 mg/dL in men, less than 50 mg/dL in women) have a higher risk of heart disease.

Heart attack (Myocardial infarction) Death of or damage to part of the heart muscle due to an insufficient blood supply when one of the coronary arteries that supply blood to the heart muscle is blocked (atherosclerotic plague). If a plaque deposit tears or ruptures, a blood clot may form and block the artery, causing a heart attack.

Heart block A condition in which electrical impulses are not conducted in the normal fashion from the atria to the ventricles caused by damage or disease processes within the cardiac conduction system.

Heart failure (Congestive heart failure) The inability of the heart to pump enough blood to meet the needs of the body's other organs causing buildup of fluid in the body, seen as swelling (edema), most commonly in the lower legs and ankles. HF may affect the right side, the left side, or both sides of the heart. Right-sided HF affects the gastrointestinal tract and the extremities and usually occurs as a result of left-sided HF. Left-sided HF affects the lungs, but as the heart's ability to pump decreases, fluid builds up in tissues throughout the body. Most areas of the body can be affected when both sides of the heart fail. The most common causes of HF are coronary artery disease (CAD), previous heart attack, and hypertension. HF becomes more common with advancing age.

Heart murmur An abnormal sound in the heart caused by defective heart valves or holes in the heart walls made by blood circulating through the heart's chambers and valves, or through blood vessels near the heart. A person can be born with a heart murmur, or it can be caused by pregnancy, fever, thyrotoxicosis, or anemia.

Heart rate Is the number of heartbeats per unit of time, typically expressed as beats per minute (bpm). A normal resting heart rate for adults range from 60 to 100 beats a minute.

Heart Transplant Surgery that replaces a damaged heart with a healthy heart taken from a donor who has been declared brain dead.

Heart valve The valves—four in the heart—control the one directional blood flow through the heart by opening and closing with each heartbeat . The four valves are: tricuspid valve (between the right atrium and the right ventricle), pulmonary valve (between the right ventricle and the pulmonary artery), mitral valve (between the left atrium and the left ventricle), and aortic valve (between the left ventricle and the aorta).

Heart valve replacement surgery (Artificial heart valve surgery) Open-heart surgery to replace a defective or diseased heart valve. Replacement heart valves are either natural (biologic) or artificial (mechanical). Natural valves are from human donors. Modified natural valves come from animal donors. Artificial valves are made of metal.

Hemodynamics The forces involved in circulating blood through the cardiovascular system. The heart adapts its hemodynamic performance to the needs of the body, increasing its output of blood when muscles are working and decreasing output when the body is at rest.

Heterograft A graft of tissue or an organ from one species to another species

Holter monitoring A technique for the continuous recording of electrocardiographic (ECG) signals, usually over 24 h, to detect and diagnose ECG changes (ambulatory monitoring).

Homocysteine An amino acid naturally found in the blood that may serve as a marker for higher risk of coronary artery disease (CAD), stroke, and peripheral vascular disease.

Homograft A graft of tissue or an organ from a donor of the same species as the recipient

Hypercholesterolemia High levels of blood cholesterol, a major risk factor for coronary heart disease, heart attack, and stroke. Target total normal cholesterol level less than 200 mg/dL

Hyperemia The increase of blood flow to different tissues in the body.

Hyperglycemia A condition with increased levels in plasma glucose (blood sugar). It can turn into a complex medical condition—diabetic ketoacidosis and coma—if it's not treated on time and adequately. A subject with a consistent range between 100 and 126 mg/dL (American Diabetes Association guidelines) is considered hyperglycemic, while above 126 mg/dL or 7 mmol/L is generally held to have diabetes.

Hyperplasia Increased cell production in a normal tissue or organ. Hyperplasia may be a sign of abnormal or precancerous changes.

Hypertension A chronic increase in blood pressure above normal range. Blood pressures of 120–139/80–89 mm Hg are considered pre-hypertension. People with pre-hypertension are likely to develop high blood pressure unless steps are taken to control blood pressure. Blood pressure is considered high if it is 140/90 mm Hg or higher; above 180/110 is considered severe.

Hypertriglyceridemia High levels of triglycerides in the blood. A high triglyceride level combined with low HDL cholesterol or high LDL cholesterol seems to speed up atherosclerosis. A normal triglyceride level is less than 150 mg/dL.

Hypertrophic cardiomyopathy Is a condition in which the heart muscle becomes thick. The thickening can make it harder for blood to leave the heart, forcing the heart to work harder to pump blood. It also can make it harder for the heart to relax and fill with blood.

Hypertrophy Is the increase in the volume of an organ or tissue due to the enlargement of its component cells.

Hypoglycemia A low level of plasma glucose. Hypoglycemia can occur after insulin excess and/or inadequate glucose intake, among other causes. These situations are common in people with diabetes who receive too much insulin or who don't eat enough. Blood sugar below 70 mg/dL is considered low.

Hypoxia Reduction of oxygen supply to a tissue below physiological levels, despite adequate perfusion of the tissue by blood (anemic hypoxia—reduction of the oxygen-carrying capacity of the blood, histotoxic hypoxia—impaired use of oxygen by tissues, hypoxic hypoxia—insufficient oxygen reaching the blood, stagnant hypoxia—failure to transport sufficient oxygen because of inadequate blood flow).

Hypoplastic left heart syndrome A congenital defect in which the left side of the heart is underdeveloped .

Hypotension The medical term for abnormally low blood pressure and is generally considered if: systolic blood pressure is less than 90 mm Hg or diastolic less than 60 mm Hg. However, in practice, blood pressure is considered too low only if evident signs are present.

Implantable cardioverter defibrillator (ICD) An internal defibrillator is used in patients at risk for recurrent, sustained ventricular tachycardia, or fibrillation. ICDs look similar to a pacemaker and are about the size of a pocket watch. ICDs run on batteries and can last many years.

Incidence The number of new cases of a disease that develop in a population during a 1-year period.

Inferior vena cava A major vein that carries blood from the lower body (legs and abdomen) to the heart.

Insulin A hormone produced in the pancreas needed to turn sugar and other food into energy.

Insufficiency (valve) Describes a condition in which a valve is not able to prevent back-flow of blood. The resulting backflow is termed regurgitation.

Intraaortic balloon pump A device used in treating severe left ventricular failure. IBP essentially assists the left ventricle to pump and increases cardiac output.

Intravascular ultrasound A medical imaging methodology using a specially designed catheter with a miniaturized ultrasound probe attached to the distal end of the catheter. This technique is particularly helpful in cases of complex narrowing (stenosis), as may occur in the aorta (coarctation) or pulmonary arteries.

Ischemia Insufficient blood flow to tissue due to blockage in the blood flow through the arteries.

Ischemic heart disease (Coronary artery disease, Coronary heart disease) Blockages in the coronary arteries lead to ischemia or decreased blood flow to the heart muscle. Symptoms of stable ischemic heart disease include characteristic chest pain on exertion and decreased exercise tolerance. Unstable IHD presents itself as chest pain or other symptoms at rest, or rapidly worsening angina.

Laser angioplasty A technique used to open coronary arteries blocked by atherosclerotic plaque. A catheter with a laser at its tip is inserted into an artery and advanced through the artery to the blockage. When the laser is in position, it emits pulsating beams of light that vaporize the plaque.

LDL cholesterol (Low-density lipoprotein) Often called "bad" cholesterol, LDL cholesterol is the major cholesterol carrier in the blood. A high level of LDL cholesterol (160 mg/dL and above) reflects an increased risk of heart disease. An optimal level is less than 100 mg/dL. Levels from 100 to 129 mg/dL are near or optimal. Levels from 130–159 mg/dL are borderline high, which also increases risk for heart disease or stroke.

Left-ventricular assist device (LVAD) A battery-operated, surgically implanted mechanical pump-type device that helps maintain the pumping ability of a heart. This device is sometimes called a "bridge to transplant," but is now used in long-term therapy.

Lipid A fatty substance insoluble in blood. Cholesterol, cholesterol compounds, and triglycerides are all lipids. They are transported in the blood as part of large molecules called lipoproteins.

List mode A method of computer data collection where x and y positional signals are stored sequentially in memory in the form of list.

Low-density lipoprotein (LDL) A type of protein that transports "bad" cholesterol in the blood. It's the major cholesterol carrier in the blood.

Lumen The open space within a tube, such as a blood vessel.

Mammary prosthesis A breast augmentation-reconstruction implant.

Maze procedure A surgical procedure to control atrial fibrillation and/or atrial flutter. A number of incisions are made in the atria to block the path of the arrhythmia.

Metabolic syndrome A name for a group of risk factors that occur together and increase the risk for coronary artery disease, stroke, and type 2 diabetes.

Minimally invasive heart surgery (MIHS) (Limited Access Coronary Artery Surgery) An alternative to standard bypass surgery (CABG). Small incisions (ports) are made in the chest. The instruments are passed through the ports to perform the bypasses. In some cases the surgeon views these operations on video monitors rather than directly.

Mirror imaging artifact A type of ultrasound artifact that may be created adjacent to a highly reflective acoustic interface.

Mitral valve A bicuspid valve that separates the left atrium and the left ventricle and prevents backflow from the ventricle to the atrium.

Mitral valve prolapse (MVP) In MVP, one or both valve flaps are enlarged, and some of their supporting "strings" may be too long. When the heart pumps (contracts), the mitral valve flaps don't close smoothly or evenly, and part of one or both flaps collapses backward into the left atrium allowing a small amount of blood leak backward through the valve.

Mitral valve stenosis Narrowing of the mitral valve limits the forward flow of blood from the heart's left upper chamber (atrium) to the left lower chamber (ventricle), causing a backup of blood and fluid in the lungs. Mitral valve stenosis most commonly develops many years after a person has had rheumatic fever.

Mortality The total number of deaths from a given disease in a population during an interval of time, usually a year.

Multiplanar reconstruction (MPR) The reformatting of images acquired in the original axial plane to produce images in either the coronal, sagittal, or oblique plane.

Myocardial biopsy (Endomyocardial biopsy) A small amount of tissue is removed from the internal lining of the heart for testing. It is used to help diagnose and treat heart muscle disorders and is also used to detect rejection of the new heart after a heart transplant.

Myocardial infarction Death of a portion of the heart muscle tissue due to a blockage or interruption in the supply of blood to the heart muscle.

Myocardial ischemia A condition in which there is not enough blood flow (and thus oxygen and nutrient supply) to the heart muscle.

Myocardial perfusion imaging (MPI) A noninvasive way to assess the blood flow to the muscle of the heart. Is also known by other names, including myocardial perfusion scan, thallium scan, sestamibi cardiac scan, and nuclear stress test.

Myocardial septum Tissue separating the heart chambers.

Myocarditis Inflammation of the heart muscle (myocardium).

Myocardium The middle and the thickest layer of the heart wall composed of cardiac muscle cells that forms the bulk of the heart wall and contracts as the organ beats. The myocardium is the layer that has the largest oxygen needs and is most affected by decreased blood flow (ischemia).

Myocytes The individual cells of the heart.

Nitroglycerin A drug that dilates blood vessels and increases the supply of blood and oxygen to the heart, while reducing its workload. Nitroglycerin spray and tablets are used to treat episodes of angina in people who have coronary artery disease.

Node Component of the electrical conductance system in the cardiac tissue.

Noise Extraneous interference in electronic circuit of statistical manipulation

Normalize A term used in association with computer-defined ROI to indicate that counts contained in the regions have been converted to the same size of region

Nyquist frequency The highest frequency that can be coded at a given sampling rate that can be represented in an image.

Obesity An excess of body fat. Obesity is defined as a body mass index (BMI) of 30.0 kg/m^2 or greater or about 30 pounds or more over ideal body weight. Extreme obesity is defined as a BMI of 40.0 kg/m^2 or more.

Occluded artery An artery in which blood flow has been impaired by a blockage.

Overweight A body mass index (BMI) of 25.0–29.9 kg/m^2. A BMI of 25 kg/m^2 corresponds to about 10 % over ideal body weight.

Pacemaker A medical device that uses electrical impulses, delivered by electrodes contacting the heart muscles, to regulate the action of the heart.

Palpitations The sensation of the heart beating rapidly or irregularly.

Paramedical Pertaining or closely related to the art or practice of medicine. This term is often applied to personnel whose work supports, or is closely related to, that of practicing physicians.

Patent ductus arteriosus (PDA) A congenital heart defect that allows blood to mix between the pulmonary artery and the aorta. Before birth an open passage way (the ductus arteriosus) exists between these two blood vessels which normally closes within a few hours of birth. When this doesn't happen, some blood that should flow through the aorta returns to the lungs

Percutaneous coronary intervention (PCI) See angioplasty

Pericardial sac The fibrous membrane surrounding the myocardium

Pericarditis A disorder caused by inflammation of the pericardium, which is the sac-like covering of the heart. It's usually a complication of a viral, bacterial, or fungal infection or can result from a heart attack, cancer, injury, or surgery.

Pericardium The outer fibrous "sac" that surrounds the heart.

Peripheral artery disease (PAD) A type of peripheral vascular disease that affects blood circulation, mainly in arteries leading to the legs and feet. Symptoms include pain in the legs or buttocks when exercising that goes away when the activity is stopped, though not everyone has symptoms. Smokers are at a much higher risk for PAD.

Peripheral vascular disease Diseases of blood vessels outside the heart and brain or diseases of the lymph vessels. Peripheral artery disease (PAD) is a common form of peripheral vascular disease.

Peritoneal jugular (LeVeen) shunt A shunt designed to drain fluid from the peritoneal cavity to the central venous system.

Pigtail Used to describe the appearance of the end of a drainage catheter or angiography catheter with a curvature similar to that of a pig's tail.

Plaque Atheroma, a cholesterol-laden buildup in the interior wall of blood vessels. The building up of plaque and hardening of the arteries is known as atherosclerosis.

Plasma lipid The lipid (fatty particles) carried in blood.

Platelets An element in blood that aids in blood clotting.

Poisson distribution A discrete frequency distribution that gives the probability of a number of independent events occurring in a fixed time

Polycythemia An elevated number of red blood cells, also referred to as a "high hematocrit" or "thick blood."

Polyunsaturated fats A type of fat found mainly in vegetable oils such as corn, safflower, sunflower, and soybean oils, as well as in seeds and fish. Polyunsaturated fats may help lower blood cholesterol levels when used in place of saturated fats.

Porcine graft (valve) A biologic body part derived from a pig.

Port-A-Cath A type of vascular access port.

Potassium (K+) One of the electrolyte substances found naturally in the body that, together with sodium and calcium, regulates the body's water balance, maintains normal heart rhythm, and is responsible for nerve impulse conduction and muscle contraction. A proper balance of potassium, sodium, calcium, and magnesium is essential for normal excitability of muscle tissue, especially cardiac muscle, and plays a role in nerve conduction. Small changes in the potassium concentration outside cells can have substantial effects on the activity of nerves and muscles.

Precision Also called reproducibility or repeatability; is the degree to which repeated measurements under unchanged conditions show the same results

Premature atrial contraction (PAC) A contraction in the atrium which is initiated by an ectopic focus and occurs earlier than the next expected normal sinus beat.

Premature ventricular contraction (PVC or VPD) A contraction in the ventricle which is initiated by an ectopic focus and occurs earlier than the next expected normal sinus or escape rhythm beat.

Prevalence The total number of cases of a given disease in a population at a specific time. Prevalence is sometimes expressed as a percentage of population.

Prolapse Floppy valve, associated with regurgitation. Mitral valve prolapse (MVP)—The valve that separates the upper and lower chambers of the left side of the heart does not close properly.

Prostaglandins One of a number of hormone-like substances that participate in a wide range of body functions such as the contraction and relaxation of smooth muscle, the dilation and constriction of blood vessels, control of blood pressure, and modulation of inflammation.

Pulmonary Relating to the lungs.

Pulmonary artery catheterization (Right heart catheterization) Used to evaluate primary pulmonary hypertension. A thin, flexible tube (called a Swan-Ganz catheter) is usually inserted in one of the veins in the neck and threaded into the right ventricle and pulmonary artery. This is a common way to measure the pressure in the pulmonary artery and find out what treatment is appropriate for a given patient. (Sometimes called Swan-Ganz Catheterization)

Pulmonary atresia A congenital heart defect in which no pulmonary valve exists. Blood can't flow from the right ventricle into the pulmonary artery and on to the lungs.

Pulmonary edema Fluid buildup in the lungs usually due to mitral stenosis or left ventricular failure. Symptoms of pulmonary edema include difficulty breathing, coughing up blood, excessive sweating, anxiety, and pale skin.

Pulmonary stenosis (PS) A congenital heart defect in which the pulmonary valve—between the right ventricle and the pulmonary artery—is defective and doesn't open properly.

Pulmonary valve A semilunar (describing the shape: half moon) valve separating the pulmonary artery and the right ventricle.

Pulmonary veins Four veins that return blood from the lungs to the heart. They empty into the left atrium.

Purkinje fibers The specialized cardiac muscle fibers, part of the impulse-conducting network of the heart, that swiftly convey impulses from the atrioventricular node to the ventricles.

Receptor A structure on the surface of a cell (or inside a cell) that selectively receives and binds a specific substance

Reentry A type of abnormal conduction in which electrical impulses get caught in a merry-go-round-like sequence. This is a common cause of tachycardias.

Regurgitation The leakage that results when a heart valve that doesn't close properly and lets blood leak back into the chamber from which it was pumped.

Reperfusion therapy One or more techniques to restore blood flow to part of the heart muscle damaged during a heart attack or part of the brain injured during a stroke. It may include clot-dissolving drugs (thrombolysis), balloon angioplasty, or surgery.

Restenosis Literally means the "re"occurrence of "stenosis," a narrowing of a blood vessel, leading to restricted blood flow. Restenosis usually relates to an artery or other large blood vessel that has become narrowed, received treatment to clear the blockage, and subsequently become again narrowed.

Retrospective reconstruction Image reconstruction after raw data have been saved, e.g., MPR and 3 D volume rendering.

Rheumatic heart disease Damage done to the heart, particularly the heart valves, by one or more attacks of rheumatic fever.

Right heart ventriculography A study of the right chambers (atrium and ventricle) of the heart. This is done by injecting contrast media through the catheter into the heart's right side with a rapid succession of X-rays taken to capture images of blood flow.

Ring artifact A type of computed tomographic artifact usually caused by a faulty detector producing rings or concentric circles on computed tomographic images.

Risk factor An element or condition involving certain hazard or danger. When referring to the heart and blood vessels, a positive risk factor is associated with an increased chance of developing cardiovascular disease including stroke. A negative risk factor is associated with a reduced chance of developing heart and blood vessel disease.

ROC curve A plot of the true positive rate against the false positive rate for the different possible cutpoints of a diagnostic test. The ROC curve is a fundamental tool for diagnostic test evaluation

Saturated fats Types of fat found in all foods from animals (i.e., butter, cheese, whole milk, ice cream, cream, and fatty meats) and from some plants (i.e., coconut, palm, and palm kernel oils). They are the biggest dietary cause of high LDL "bad" cholesterol levels. Limit any foods that are high (e.g., over 20 %) in saturated fat. Limit saturated fat intake to 7–10 % of total calories (or less) each day.

Sensitivity Measures the proportion of actual positives which are correctly identified as such (e.g., the percentage of sick people who are correctly identified as having the condition)

Septum The muscular wall dividing the chambers on the heart's left side from the chambers on the right

Shunt (1) An abnormal flow pattern of blood through the chambers of the heart or through the large arteries leaving the heart. A "left-to-right" shunt results in extra blood flow entering the lungs, while a "right-to-left" shunt results in decreased blood flow to the lungs, low oxygen levels, and cyanosis. (2) A surgically created connection designed to increase the delivery of blood to the lungs.

Silent ischemia Episodes of ischemia that aren't accompanied by pain.

Single photon emission computed tomography (SPECT) A nuclear imaging technique that involves injecting a radioactive liquid into the blood, and then acquiring multiple 2-D images (projections), from multiple angles. A computer processing is used to apply a tomographic reconstruction algorithm to the multiple projections, yielding a 3-D dataset.

Sinoatrial (SA) node The heart's natural pacemaker located in the right atrium. Electrical impulses originate here and travel through the heart, causing it to beat.

Sinogram A two-dimensional projection space representation of a transaxial image where one dimension refers to radial distance from the center, and the second dimension refers to projection angle.

Sinus rhythm The normal heart rate and rhythm of the heart. The heart rate during normal sinus rhythm is 60–100 beats per minute (BPM).

Sodium (Na) A mineral that, together with potassium and calcium, regulates the body's water balance, maintains normal heart rhythm, and is responsible for nerve impulse conduction and muscle contraction. In people who already have high blood pressure, too much sodium may increase the risk of stroke, heart disease, and kidney damage. Table salt (sodium chloride) is 40 % sodium. Recommended intake of sodium is less than 1,500 mg per day

Spasm The sudden, temporary, or prolonged contraction of a muscle or artery.

Specificity Measures the proportion of negatives which are correctly identified (e.g., the percentage of healthy people who are correctly identified as not having the condition).

Sphygmomanometer (Blood pressure monitor) An instrument for measuring blood pressure.

Stable angina Predictable chest discomfort that usually occurs during exertion or under mental or emotional stress.

Stages of heart failure Developed by the American Heart Association and the American College of Cardiology in 2001. Stages A and B represent people who have not yet developed heart failure, but are at high risk to do so because of coronary artery disease (CAD), high blood pressure, diabetes, or other predisposing risk factor. Stage C includes patients with past or current symptoms of heart failure who have structural heart disease. Stage D includes patients who have advanced heart failure that is difficult to manage with standard treatment.

Standard deviation The square root of the variance where variance is the average of the squared differences from the Mean

Statins A group of drugs used to reduce elevated low-density lipoprotein (LDL) or "bad" cholesterol, which is associated with increased risk of cardiovascular disease. They work in the liver to prevent cholesterol from forming. They are also known as HMG CoA reductase inhibitors. Atorvastatin (Lipitor), lovastatin (Mevacor), pravastatin (Pravachol), rosuvastatin (Crestor), and simvastatin (Zocor) are examples of statins.

Stenosis Constriction of a passage. Used typically when there is a narrowing of a valve opening (e.g., mitral valve stenosis) or of a blood vessel.

Stent A small mesh tube that's used to treat narrow or weak arteries.

Stent procedure Using a wire mesh tube (a stent) to prop open an artery that's recently been cleared using angioplasty.

Stethoscope An instrument for listening to sounds within the body.

Stress Bodily or mental tension resulting from a person's response to physical, chemical, or emotional factors. Stress can refer to physical exertion as well as mental anxiety.

Stress test A test used in medicine and cardiology to measure the heart's ability to respond to exercise or pharmacological intervention in a controlled environment.

Subaortic stenosis A congenital heart defect in which the left ventricle is narrowed (stenosis) just below the aortic valve, which blood passes through to go into the aorta.

Sudden cardiac death (SCD) Death due to cardiac causes within 1 h of the onset of symptoms, with no prior warning—usually caused by ventricular fibrillation.

Superior vena cava A major vein that carries blood from the upper body (head, neck, chest, and arms) to the heart.

Supraventricular tachycardia A condition originating from above the ventricles in which heart tissue in either the upper chambers (atria) or the middle region (above the ventricles) develops pacemaker activity, resulting in an abnormally fast heartbeat.

Swan-Ganz catheter A soft catheter with an expandable balloon tip that is used for measuring blood pressure in the pulmonary artery, named for its inventors, Jeremy Swan and William Ganz. (See Pulmonary Artery Catheterization)

Syncope Passing out, loss of consciousness, or fainting which may be caused by a temporary deficiency of oxygen in the brain.

Systole The contraction phase of the normal heart cycle during which blood is driven into the aorta and pulmonary artery.

Systolic blood pressure The highest blood pressure measured in the arteries. It is measured in millimeters of mercury (mmHg), and is the upper number in the standard blood pressure reading.

Systolic heart failure A condition in which the heart pumps with less strength than normal (decreased ejection fraction). This type of heart failure is more common and caused by coronary artery disease (CAD), high blood pressure, valvular heart disease, and idiopathic cardiomyopathy.

Tachycardia (Tachyarrhythmia) Rapid beating of either or both chambers of the heart, usually defined as a rate over 100 beats per minute.

Tetralogy of Fallot A complex, congenital heart defect with four components: ventricular septal defect, pulmonary valve stenosis, muscular right ventricle, and the aorta directly over the ventricular septal defect.

Thallium stress test A type of nuclear scanning test similar to a routine exercise stress test but with images. The radionuclide tracers sestamibi and tetrofosmin can also be used instead of thallium for this test. (Also known as Myocardial Perfusion Imaging (MPI), Radionuclide Stress Test, and Nuclear Stress Test.)

Thoracostomy tube Used to drain pleural fluid collections or reexpand the lung in cases of a pneumothorax (chest tube).

Thrombolysis The breaking up of a blood clot.

Thrombosis The formation or presence of a blood clot (thrombus) inside a blood vessel or chamber of the heart.

Thrombus A blood clot that forms inside a blood vessel or chamber of the heart

Tracheostomy tube A tube directly inserted into the trachea through the anterior tracheal cartilage.

Trans fats (Trans fatty acids) A fat that is formed when liquid vegetable oils go through a chemical process called hydrogenation in which hydrogen is added to make the oils more solid. Hydrogenated vegetable fats are used by food processors because they allow longer shelf life and give food desirable taste, shape, and texture. The majority of trans fat can be found in shortenings, stick (or hard) margarine, cookies, crackers, snack foods, fried foods (including fried fast food), doughnuts, pastries, baked goods, and other processed foods made with or fried in partially hydrogenated oils. Evidence suggests that consuming trans fat can raise LDL ("bad) cholesterol levels and lower HDL ("good") cholesterol levels.

Transesophageal echocardiography (TEE) An ultrasound technique in which the ultrasound probe is placed in the esophagus to "look" at the heart from behind. TEE is much more sensitive than transthoracic (across the chest) echocardiography, as overlying structures (bone and lungs) do not obscure the view.

Transient ischemic attack (TIA) A "mini stroke," TIA is caused by a temporary disturbance of blood supply to an area of the brain and it lasts for only for a short time. TIA is an extremely important indicator of future stroke.

Transmyocardial revascularization (TMR) Laser procedure used to relieve severe angina or chest pain in very ill patients who aren't candidates for bypass surgery or angioplasty. The laser may stimulate new blood vessels to grow, called angiogenesis, or it may destroy nerve fibers to the heart, making patients unable to feel their chest pain.

Transposition of the great arteries A congenital heart defect in which the positions of the pulmonary artery and the aorta are reversed. The aorta receives the oxygen-poor blood from the right ventricle, but it's carried back to the body without receiving more oxygen. Likewise, the pulmonary artery receives the oxygen-rich blood from the left ventricle, but carries it back to the lungs.

Tricuspid atresia A congenital heart defect in which there's no tricuspid valve. That means no blood can flow from the right atrium to the right ventricle, and as a result, the right ventricle is small and not fully developed.

Tricuspid valve Valve that separates the right atrium and the right ventricle and prevents backflow from the ventricle to the atrium. It is composed of three leaf-like parts.

Triglycerides The chemical form in which most fat exists in food, as well as in the body. They're also present in blood plasma, and, in association with cholesterol, form the plasma lipids. They can be made in the body from energy sources such as carbohydrates or come from fats eaten in foods. The normal level of triglycerides is less than 150 mg/dL. Excess triglycerides have been linked to the occurrence of coronary artery disease (CAD).

Troponins Proteins found in heart muscle. Cardiac troponin T and troponin I are the most specific and sensitive laboratory markers of myocardial cell injury, and therefore have replaced creatine kinase MB as the gold standard.

Truncus arteriosus A complex congenital heart defect where only one artery arises from the heart and forms the aorta and pulmonary artery. Surgery for this condition usually is required early in life. Children with truncus arteriosus need lifelong follow-up to see how well the heart is working. People with truncus arteriosus, before and after treatment, are at risk for getting an infection on the heart's walls or valves (endocarditis). It is recommended that all people with uncorrected or partially corrected truncus arteriosus take antibiotics before certain dental procedures. If you (or your child) have had corrective surgery, ask your cardiologist whether there is still a need for these routineantibiotics.

T-tube drain A type of traditional gravity drain configured in a T shape. T-tubes are most often used for common bile duct drainage.

Type 1 diabetes Insulin-dependent diabetes (IDDM). A condition characterized by high blood glucose levels caused by a total lack of insulin. It can occur at any age but is usually diagnosed in children and young adults.

Type 2 diabetes The most common form of diabetes: noninsulin-dependent diabetes (NIDDM). Type 2 diabetes occurs in two ways: (1) The body does not create enough insulin or (2) The body cannot use the insulin efficiently. Patients with type 2 diabetes are faced with the daily challenge of controlling blood glucose levels to prevent or delay the onset of many serious life-threatening health complications such as cardiovascular disease.

Ultrasound High-frequency sound vibrations, not audible to the human ear, used in medical diagnosis.

Unstable angina Chest pain or discomfort that's unexpected and usually occurs while at rest. The discomfort may be more severe and prolonged than typical angina or be the first time a person has angina. Unstable angina is an acute coronary syndrome and should be treated as an emergency.

Valve A one-way flap preventing the backflow of blood. There are four valves in the heart.

Vascular Referring to the vessels

Vasoconstriction A narrowing of a blood vessel, causing decreased blood flow to a part of the body.

Vasodilators A group of drugs that cause the muscle in the walls of the blood vessels (especially the arterioles) to relax, allowing the vessels to dilate. Nitroglycerin is a vasodilator.

Vein Carries blood, mostly deoxygenated, from the tissues to the heart. The pulmonary vein is the only one to carry oxygenated blood, which is from the lungs to the heart.

Vena cava The veins that empty directly into the right atrium, known as the superior and inferior vena cava.

Ventricle The larger two chambers in the lower portion of the heart, known as the right and left ventricle separated by the interventricular septum; valves separate the ventricles from the pulmonary artery (right) and aorta (left).

Ventricular assist device (VAD) A device used to assist the heart in its blood pumping function (univentricular or biventricular)

Ventricular fibrillation (VF) Very fast, chaotic, quivering heart contractions that start in the ventricles. If left untreated, it may result in cardiac arrest. The most common cause of VF is a heart attack, but VF can occur whenever the heart muscle is affected by a poor supply of oxygen (ischemia) or by specific heart disorders. Death will occur if defibrillation is not initiated within 6 min from the onset of VF.

Ventricular systole Contraction of the ventricles, pushing blood into the lungs and aorta

Ventricular tachycardia (VT) A rapid heart rate that starts in the ventricles. During VT, the heart does not have time to fill with enough blood between heart beats to supply the entire body with sufficient blood. It may cause dizziness and light-headedness.

Ventricular septal defect (VSD) The most common congenital heart defect in which one or more holes exist in the muscular wall that separates the heart's right and left ventricles.

Ventriculoperitoneal shunt A shunt system designed to reduce intracranial pressure and prevent the development of hydrocephalus

Venules Small veins, the blood vessels that carry blood back to the heart and lungs.

Windowing The process of selecting some segment of the total pixel value range and then displaying the pixel values within that segment over the full brightness (shades of gray) range from white to black

Wolff–Parkinson–White Syndrome (WPW) A condition in which the heart beats too fast due to abnormal, extra electrical pathways between the heart's upper and lower chambers. WPW can be present at birth but symptoms can appear at any time. More women than men are diagnosed with WPW. Treatments include medications and some surgical procedures.

Xenograft Same as a heterograft

Z-stent A generic term for a variety of metallic stents used to overcome areas of narrowing in such tubular structures as vessels, bile ducts, ureters, and the urethra.

Appendix C
Useful Websites

PubMedHealth http://www.ncbi.nlm.nih.gov/pubmedhealth
ACR American College of Radiology http://www.acr.org/
AHA http://www.heart.org/
Amedeo. The Medical Literature Guide http://www.amedeo.com/
American AED/CPR Association http://www.aedcpr.com/
ARRT American Registry of Radiologic Technologists https://www.arrt.org/index.html
ASRT American Society of Radiologic Technologists https://www.asrt.org/
ASNC American Society of Nuclear Cardiology http://www.asnc.org/
AuntMinnie.com http://www.auntminnie.com/
Author Stream (slide sharing) http://www.authorstream.com
Basic Heart Terminology http://suite101.com/article/basic-heart-terminology-a149641
Cardiac Care Critique http://www.cardiaccarecritique.com/products/petct/petct.php#
Cardiovascular Physiology Concepts http://www.cvphysiology.com
CathLabDigest http://www.cathlabdigest.com/articles/Angiographic-Projections-Made-Simple-Easy-Guide-Understanding-Oblique-Views
CDC Centers for Disease Control http://www.cdc.gov/
Clinical Key Elsevier https://www.clinicalkey.com/
Consultants in Nuclear Medicine http://www.nucmedconsultants.com/
Dose Estimates for Nuclear Medicine Scans http://ehs.columbia.edu/Dosimetry%20Help/NMDoseEstimates.html
DOT Department of Transportation http://www.dot.gov/
Drugs.com http://www.drugs.com/
ECG Teacher http://ecgteacher.com/
Emedicine http://emedicine.medscape.com
EPA Environmental Protection Agency http://www.epa.gov/
Family Health Guide. Harvard Medical School. http://www.health.harvard.edu/fhg/
FDA *Food and Drug Administration* http://www.fda.gov/
HFAP Healthcare Facilities Accreditation Program http://www.hfap.org/
HPS. Health Physics Society http://www.hps.org/
GE (General Electric) Healthcare https://hls.gehealthcare.com/gehc/

A. Moniuszko and B.A. Kesala, *Nuclear Cardiology Study Guide: A Technologist's Review for Passing Specialty Certification Exams*, DOI 10.1007/978-1-4614-8645-9, © Springer Science+Business Media New York 2014

HealthImaging.com http://www.healthimaging.com/
ICANL *Intersocietal Commission for the Accreditation of Nuclear Medicine Laboratories* http://www.icanl.org/icanl/index.htm
ICRP International Commission on Radiological Protection http://www.icrp.org/
ICRU International Commission on Radiation Units http://www.icru.org/
IAEA International Atomic Energy Agency http://www.iaea.org/
Image wisely http://imagewisely.org/
IMAIOSE E-anatomy http://www.imaios.com/en/e-Anatomy/
Internet Journal of Nuclear Medicine http://www.ispub.com/ostia/index.php?xml FilePath=journals/ijnuc/vol3n1/scan.xml
Jefferson Lab http://www.jlab.org/div_dept/train/rad_guide/effects.html
JCAHO Joint Commission on Accreditation of Healthcare Organizations http://www.jointcommission.org/
Journal of Nuclear Cardiology http://www.onlinejnc.com/index.html
Mallinckrodt Inst of Radiology WU in St Louis Teaching file. http://gamma.wustl.edu/
Mallinckrodt Institute of Radiology cases http://www.radquiz.com/Nucs-Teaching.htm
MDConsult http://www.mdconsult.com
MDS Nordion http://www.mds.nordion.com/
Medical Physics Dep, http://www.nuclearmedicine.org.uk/ Pilgrim Hosp, Boston
Medscape http://www.medscape.com/
MollecularImaging http://www.molecularimaging.net/
North American Center for Continuing Medical Education http://www.naccme.com/
NCBI. PubMed.gov National Center for Biotechnology Information http://www.ncbi.nlm.nih.gov/pubmed/
NCI National Cancer Institute http://www.cancer.gov/
NCRP National Council on Radiation Protection & Measurements http://www.ncrponline.org/
NEMA National Electrical Manufacturer's Association http://www.nema.org/
North American Center for Continuing Medical Education http://www.naccme.com/
Nuclear Medical Tutorials http://www.nucmedtutorials.com/
Nuclear Medicine. Radiochemistry Society. http://www.radiochemistry.org/nuclearmedicine/
Nuclear Medicine Technology Certification Board http://www.nmtcb.org/root/default.php
Oxford Journals. Radiation Protection Dosimetry http://rpd.oxfordjournals.org/content/
Philips http://www.healthcare.philips.com/
Quality Assurance in Gamma Camera & SPECT Systems http://www.medphysics.wisc.edu/courses/mp573/NM%3FPET%20radlab/HalamaSlides.pdf
RADAR RAdiation Dose Assessment Resource www.doseinforadar.com
RADAR Patient Exposure Radiation Dose Calculator http://www.doseinfo-radar.com/ExposureCalculator.html.
RadiologyInfo.org http://www.radiologyinfo.org/
Radiological Society of North America (USA) http://www.rsna.org
Radiopharmacy, Inc. http://www.radiopharmacy.com/Newsletters.htm

REMM Radiation Emergency Medical Management http://www.remm.nlm.gov/dictionary.htm

RSNA Radiological Society of North America http://www.rsna.org/

Nuclear Cardiology Seminars http://www.nuclearcardiologyseminars.net/index.htm

Siemens http://www.medical.siemens.com/

SNM Society of Nuclear Medicine http://www.snm.org/

SNM. Procedure guideline for the use of radiopharmaceuticals 4.0. http://www.snm.org/guidelines

Societies of Nuclear Medicine of Latin America http://www.alasbimnjournal.cl/

UpToDate http://www.uptodate.com/home/

U.S. NRC *Nuclear Regulatory Commission* http://www.nrc.gov/

U.S. NRC *Nuclear Regulatory Commission*. NRC Regulations, Title 10, Code of Federal Regulations. http://www.nrc.gov/reading-rm/doc-collections/cfr/

WIKIPEDIA http://www.wikipedia.org/

Index

A. Moniuszko and B.A. Kesala, *Nuclear Cardiology Study Guide: A Technologist's
Review for Passing Specialty Certification Exams*, DOI 10.1007/978-1-4614-8645-9,
© Springer Science+Business Media New York 2014

The manufacturer's authorised representative in the EU is Springer
Nature Customer Service Centre GmbH, Europaplatz 3, 69115 Heidelberg,
Germany. If you have any concerns regarding our products, please
contact ProductSafety@springernature.com

Printed and bound by CPI Group (UK) Ltd, Croydon, CR0 4YY
23/04/2026
02095602-0003